5/5

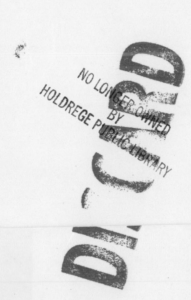

The Mandells'
IT'S NOT YOUR FAULT
YOU'RE FAT DIET

The Mandells'

IT'S
NOT
YOUR
FAULT
YOU'RE
FAT
DIET

Marshall Mandell, M.D. and
Fran Gare Mandell, M.S.

Edited by Julie Weiner

1817

HARPER & ROW, PUBLISHERS, New York

Cambridge, Philadelphia, San Francisco,
London, Mexico City, São Paulo, Sydney

Grateful acknowledgment is made for permission to reprint:

"Common Sources of Hidden Food Allergens" chart from *Dr. Mandell's Allergy-Free Cookbook* by Marshall Mandell and Fran Gare. Reprinted by permission of Marfran Publications, Inc.

FIRST EDITION

Designer: C. Linda Dingler

Library of Congress Cataloging in Publication Data

Mandell, Marshall.
   The Mandells' It's not your fault you're fat diet.

   1. Reducing diets. 2. Obesity—Nutritional aspects.
3. Food allergy.   I. Mandell, Fran Gare.   II. Weiner, Julie.   III. Title.
RM222.2.M325   1983   613.2'5   82–48124
ISBN 0–06–015114–5

83 84 85 86 87 10 9 8 7 6 5 4 3 2 1

As always, this book is dedicated to our family.

Our children, Jamie and Mark Gaberman, Steven and Nori Mandell, and David and Marc Gare.

Our grandchildren, Lane and Brian Gaberman.

To the memory of Alan Mandell, Beatrice and Albert Mandell, and David Rhein.

Most of all, this book is dedicated to Fran's mother, Henrietta Rhein, who has given us constant encouragement and love through the years. She even came from Florida to cook for us while we were writing the book, to be very sure that we would not go off the diet. Thank you, mom. We love you.

CONTENTS

Acknowledgments   ix

1. Compulsive Eating Is Not Neurotic Behavior   1
2. The Weighty Problem of Water Retention   13
3. Dr. Mandell Discusses the Allergy-Overweight
   Connection   21
4. The Psychological Advantages of the It's Not Your
   Fault You're Fat Diet   38
5. Will All Allergic-Compulsive Eaters Please
   Identify Themselves   45
6. How the Diet Works   71
7. Preparing for the Diet   79
8. The It's Not Your Fault You're Fat Diet   92
9. Every Meal's a Test Meal: The Quick Weight
   Loss Diet   151
10. Maintenance   165
11. Tips   169
12. Questions and Answers   177

Appendix A   194
Appendix B   195

Appendix C   196

Appendix D   197

Appendix E   203

Appendix F   205

Suggested Reading   209

ACKNOWLEDGMENTS

Our deepest gratitude for the invaluable assistance rendered by Julie Weiner, who helped us organize the book, conducted patient interviews, and with great competence edited the final manuscript. We thank her for her creative ideas, dedication, enthusiasm, imagination, and support along the way.

Our heartfelt thanks to our conscientious, devoted, and respected Diana Papazian, R.N., head nurse at the Alan Mandell Center for Bio-ecologic Diseases. Diana's clear thinking, accurate observations, well-kept records, and efficient help were a great contribution to the book.

A warm, all-encompassing thank-you to our entire staff at the Center: to Ester Knablin, Adrienne Gianetti, and Nan Gallicco, in Testing; Mollie Spau in the "lab"; Ellen Kates, R.N., and Melanie Rahn in Treatment; MaryBeth Lehotsky and Florence Arcamone in Administration and Reception. Because all of you care so much and give your best, our patients are getting well.

We are indebted to the patients that Julie interviewed who were so anxious to help others by sharing their experiences and suggestions. Their enthusiasm and cooperation are greatly appreciated.

A special word of thanks to Joan Jewell, Marshall's indispensable executive secretary, for quietly and efficiently "doing everything" and making it possible for him to continue with all of his many projects as well as devote so much of his time to the preparation of this book. Her input was invaluable.

We are very grateful to Faye Lustig, our innovative, industrious dynamo. As the health administrator for our Center, she kept things running smoothly in the midst of all this activity.

To Connie Clausen, a dear friend and the best agent in the publishing field—we thank you for your wisdom and help.

A special thank-you to Estherelka Kaplan, whom we are about to adopt for her continued interest, moral support, and excellent suggestions.

A thank-you, too, to Sue Battley for her editorial typing—a good job much appreciated.

And to our much loved Elda Fleurenvil; we are very pleased that you were there, keeping the house running smoothly while all of this was going on—and smiling, too.

We also want to thank our editors at Harper & Row: Lawrence Peel Ashmead and Craig D. Nelson, and our copy editors Dolores Simon, Brenda Goldberg, and Alice Huberman.

Marshall would like to express his affection, respect, and deep gratitude to his kind and wise mentor and fellow truth-seeker, Dr. Theron G. Randolph, M.D., of Chicago, the trail-blazing father of clinical ecology and modest giant among physicians. His original observations, painstaking research, brilliant concepts, and illuminating teaching on the many facets of ecologic illness and food allergy are the cornerstone of this book. Marshall also is indebted to Herbert J. Rinkel, M.D., who conceived the Rotary Diversified Diet, which you will very soon come to appreciate as an invaluable diagnostic tool that also makes it possible to successfully treat and prevent food allergies. A warm and friendly thank-you, too, to Harris Hosen, M.D., of Port Arthur, Texas, who, with his usual enthusiasm, generously shared the results of his clinical research.

The Mandells'
IT'S NOT YOUR FAULT
YOU'RE FAT DIET

1

COMPULSIVE EATING IS NOT NEUROTIC BEHAVIOR

We know what some of you are thinking: "Here we go again—another diet book, another fad diet, another gimmick, and this time they're telling me it's not my fault I'm fat. Clever, aren't they?"

No, and yes.

No, this is not just another diet book, and, no, the principles on which it is based are not some gimmick. This book is the result of forty years of research in the field of allergy and food addiction and many thousands of people tested and successfully treated, not only for overweight but for arthritis, colitis, headaches, fatigue, restlessness, nervousness, irritability, depression, bloating, indigestion, constipation, diarrhea, itching, insomnia, and many other physical, mental, emotional, and behavioral disorders which are frequently misdiagnosed as psychosomatic.

Yes, this is a diet for better health in many ways, and, yes, from it you will certainly learn that it's not your fault you're fat—or nervous, or many of the other things you have been suffering from or accusing yourself of. And, yes, simply reading these pages and going on this diet will enable you to lose many of your unwanted pounds and will probably help with many of your health problems. So don't be surprised when you find yourself with much more energy, calm, "regular," sleeping well at night, happier, and thinner—much thinner. Give us a week of your time and we will help you make some very important changes in your life.

WHAT IS ALLERGY?

Allergy is traditionally defined as an uncomfortable reaction due to a sensitivity to foods, pollens, molds, house dust, animal dander, bacteria, insect bites, or chemicals taken into the body. If a person is sensitive to them, these substances cause an allergic reaction in the body. The majority of physicians and the general public share the belief that most allergic reactions occur in the form of skin conditions, respiratory or intestinal disorders, or as a swelling reaction to an insect sting.

But in the 1940s, two trail-blazing physicians, Drs. Theron G. Randolph and Herbert J. Rinkel, advanced the field of allergy with startling new findings. They found that people could be both allergic and addicted to any substance in their diet; and if they were allergic or sensitive to something they ate, it could affect any part of their bodies and any function of their bodies, not just the classical allergic sites—skin, eyes, ears, nose, throat, bronchial tubes, and intestinal tract—as previously thought.

To understand how this can happen, think of the intestinal tract as a long passage from the mouth clear through the body. When you eat a food or drink a beverage, it enters the intestinal tract and, from there on, it has contact with every part of your body as the food is broken down in the digestive process, absorbed through the intestinal walls, and passes into the bloodstream, which then carries it to every part of the body—including the brain, which has a very rich blood supply. As a result, if you are sensitive to a food you have eaten, it could cause an allergic reaction anywhere in your body—ranging from joint pain in your fingers, knees, or hips; to stomach pain; to different kinds of malfunctions in your brain. Your muscles could react with flu-like aches, pains, or spasms (similar to palsy); your joint pain could resemble arthritis; and your brain reaction could be depression, anxiety, irritability, headache, or even schizophrenia.

At our medical center in Norwalk, Connecticut, we study and treat people with advanced and complex forms of allergic disorders. After studying 4,000-plus patients, we are no longer surprised by any physical, mental, behavioral, or "psychosomatic" disorders of children and adults caused by bodywide allergy. The name of our medical center is the Alan Mandell Center for Bio-ecologic Diseases.

Alan Mandell was my husband's oldest son, who died early in his life. Marshall believes that he could have saved Alan if he had known twenty years ago what he and his colleagues know today about nutrition and brain and body allergy. He now knows that Alan was a victim of his diet and his environment.

When Marshall speaks of the environment, he is not referring to an emotional environment, although he recognizes that this is very important: we all need support from those around us. But what Marshall and his fellow ecologists call "environment" is a physical entity. It is the house you live in and just about everything in it: the automobile you drive, your workplace, and, very important, the air you breathe, the water you drink, and the foods you eat.

At the Center, we learn from our patients. We listen to them very carefully because it is what they say about their environment and how it affects them that often tells us how to help them. We want to know everything about what they eat and breathe. That is why Marshall named his medical facility the Center for Bio-ecologic Diseases, a term Marshall coined in 1973 that means seeing the biology, genetics, physiology, and biochemistry of the body (bio) as it reacts to its environment (ecologic).

You may be thinking, "That's very interesting, but what does it have to do with the fifteen pounds I want to lose?" The answer is, "Plenty!"

What he found in most instances was that when people began to control the illness-causing factors in their environment (airborne allergens, indoor-outdoor air pollutants, chemical agents in their food and water, and the food they ate), there were important beneficial changes in their overall health. The anxious became calm, the insomniac slept, and the depressed became happy. So did the exhausted become energetic, the puffy become flat; colitis was replaced with normal bowel function; the pain of arthritis was relieved; and joint movement increased. And the obese became thin! All systems became more normal.

With our diet, most of you will not have to count calories or carbohydrates to lose weight and become healthier. As a matter of fact, you will be able to eat many kinds of food and good-size portions of them. The secret of our diet is not only the specific foods you eat but the special pattern and carefully planned frequency in which you eat them.

WE CAN BECOME ADDICTED TO FOOD

A food eaten once a day or even once every two or three days is a food you can and very well may have become addicted to. We don't know exactly why this allergic addiction develops, but there are several possible answers. One idea is that allergic addiction comes from overexposure to a food that you are allergic to without realizing it because you do not experience uncomfortable reactions immediately after eating the food and you do not link those symptoms with that food. Marshall and several other authorities on food allergy feel that food addiction may occur because the body gradually becomes sensitive to—and consequently addicted to—foods it is required to digest, absorb, and metabolize constantly, day in and day out.

Interestingly, it has been found that the kinds of foods that cause addictions vary from culture to culture, from family to family. If a family sits down to a dinner of pasta every night, with chunks of bread, and finishes with cake, they are all getting what may be for one or more of them an intolerable wheat overload. Many families have a very heavy exposure to beef and potatoes, or rice. "Health food" families might have problems with frequently eaten peanut butter, tofu (soy curds), brewer's yeast, or cereal grains. The mother of one woman Marshall treated was convinced of the importance of whole-wheat bread, so her growing daughter ate it at every meal—and ended up addictively allergic to wheat. Those of us who are or have been junk-food junkies at any time of our lives have to suspect cane sugar, corn syrup, corn starch, chocolate, wheat, yeast, milk, soy, and a host of artificial colors, flavors, and other chemical agents in these foods as the cause of our uncontrollable addictive behavior.

OUR FOOD ENVIRONMENT

Junk food introduces an important area of food allergy because sugar-loaded junk food is not just food; it is refined and processed food that contains many types of chemicals. Eating these chemicals can be a serious health hazard because they, too, pass into our bloodstreams from the digestive tract and are carried by the blood to every part of our bodies. Some of the more serious cases of addictive allergy are caused by addictions to many common food-and-chemical mixtures.

Chemical contamination of our food supply is difficult to avoid. We consume chemicals when we eat commercially grown fruits and vegetables (they have been sprayed with chemicals). Our livestock graze on chemically fertilized land, eat chemical feed, and are injected with chemicals. Fish share their waters with the chemical wastes from farming and industry. It is almost impossible to avoid them completely, but we must lessen our contact with them as much as we can. We are finding that some patients' overweight is caused by their sensitivity to chemicals. And the chemicals we eat are only one side of the environmental chemical coin; the other side is the chemical odors and fumes we breathe, because they, too, enter the bloodstream, through the lungs, and affect the body in much the same way as the chemicals we eat and drink. We see hundreds of people each year who are sensitive to various chemical substances in our food and water supply as well as to fumes that pollute the indoor and outdoor air. Many of them report that they are eating compulsively or get puffy as a result of exposure to various chemicals.

This is not allergy as traditional allergists view it but is an important form of sensitivity that seriously affects the physical and mental health of millions of chemically sensitive individuals. People with the common forms of allergy are very often the victims of chemical sensitivity, and all allergists should know how to care for them properly. Failure to take care of chemical problems can lead to treatment failures that often get blamed on patients, who may be referred to as "treatment resistant."

As a matter of fact, I, Fran, am a perfect example of moderately severe chemical sensitivity. I became depressed and ate compulsively when I was exposed to leaking natural gas. Finding out that it was the gas and not a "traumatic personality disorder" made a huge difference in my life. First of all, it was a relief to admit that I was eating compulsively after hundreds of pounds gained and lost and just as many excuses. I had blamed my mother, my former husband, my children, and my thyroid. All of my overeating, I thought, was caused by deep psychological problems, rendering me incapable of coping. As a result of these assumed problems, I couldn't resist the gratification of food. Food was enjoyable. I was convinced that eating made me feel better.

The only problem was that there were many times when I really didn't enjoy what I ate. Actually, half the time I didn't even know I had eaten it. Even so, I had my favorites. Ice cream was at the top of my list. When I started to eat ice cream, I couldn't stop until I finished every drop in the house. Heaven forbid there was a sale on half-gallons! When I finished it, I couldn't believe I had eaten "the whole thing!" Where was I while I was eating it? It wasn't until I met Marshall that I found out.

One day during the time that Marshall and I were dating, he arrived at my New York apartment to pick me up for an evening out and, instead of finding me dressed and ready, found me sitting at my kitchen table eating a pint of ice cream and crying. Any other prospective husband would have run. Instead, he became a detective. Smelling the odor of cooking gas in the apartment and knowing that what he was witnessing was not my usual behavior, he set out to find the cause. He asked me if I knew what I was doing—and I became furious. He began to check each of the apartments on my floor of the building. After knocking on several doors, he found that there was a gas leak in the supermarket that was a part of the building. He reported it to the police and fire departments and quickly forced me to leave the building. After ten minutes outdoors, I was a different person—the anger was gone, and I felt ridiculous.

This incident was my first clue that it was not my fault I was fat. I was amazed to find that a gas leak could make me both hungry and depressed. How about you? Do you have a similar story? Some of the patients who come to our Center have had similar things happen to them. They come to us having read Marshall's book, or having seen him or heard him on TV or radio, and they suspect that their problems are biologic or organic, not psychological, and are linked to some factor in their environment—like food or chemicals—not to their psyche. We usually prove them right.

DIESEL FUMES MADE HER FAT

Linda Beckwith is a perfect example of this. One of our most successful weight-loss patients, Linda lost 70 pounds and changed almost beyond recognition. One of her major chemical sensitivities is to a petroleum fraction, diesel fuel. Linda says that she is a third-generation Gypsy. She and her husband travel as much as they can. Linda told us: "As we travel around, a funny thing happens whenever we drive through a city and I start to get a good dose of diesel: By the time we get to the other end of the city, I'm famished. Not hungry, not starved—I am like an escapee from a concentration camp. *It's the kind of hunger that has no rheostat on it at all.* I'll be totally famished, even while I'm eating, until I hit the point of Thanksgiving-turkey-dinner-stuffed. I'll eat fullbore until all of a sudden I'm so stuffed that I can't move, and that's the stopping point. There's no graduation in there whatsoever as there is normally when I eat like a regular person."

Linda says it better than we ever could. That is exactly what an extreme case of compulsive eating caused by a chemical (or food) addiction is like. It comes out of the blue and stays until it can no longer be satisfied, and with it come many unwanted pounds. If you are not aware of having a chemical/food addiction, you could spend your travel life eating your way from coast to coast, feeling sure all the way that you are hungry, for every possible reason but the correct one.

Chemicals you breathe are not limited only to diesel fuel. You can have the same reaction from breathing in household cleaners, air fresheners, insecticides, paints, cosmetics—almost anything that has a "chemical" odor, like petroleum distillates and reactive substances such as ammonia, sulfur, or chlorine. So you see, chemicals that you may be susceptible to are all around you, and, like many of us, you may have been their victim without even knowing it.

It is easy to understand from my story and from Linda's how exposure to environmental chemicals often triggers irresistible biologic cravings that can completely overwhelm you and cause you to eat great quantities of unneeded foods that you never would have eaten if your system were not totally out of control. Being uncontrollably drawn to certain foods is compulsive eating and may cause food binging. The roots of these behaviors are not psychological. They arise from powerful, allergy-provoked biologic needs that you and most physicians have been totally unaware of.

DR. MANDELL DEFINES COMPULSIVE EATING

Compulsive eating comes in two forms. There are the compulsive eaters whose uncontrollable hunger or irresistible craving for certain foods is so strong that it overrides their common sense and sincere desire to lose weight. We call them the "overt compulsive eaters." Their eating problem is obvious to them, their families, and all of their friends, but the nature of the problem is not.

The second kind of compulsive eating is more subtle. Its victims are the "hidden compulsive eaters." These people have become accustomed to a certain diet of foods they are addicted to, which they eat over and over again in quantities that exceed their needs. They often do not know they are overeating and go on blissfully eating away and gaining weight totally unaware of the underlying allergic nature of their problem.

Neither of these conditions indicates that you lack willpower or that you are undisciplined. They have nothing to do with "weak moral fiber." Nothing!

At the Center, I have found that almost every case of compulsive eating has an allergic basis. It is called "addictive food allergy." That's right—addictive. Foods and chemicals can be addictive, much the way food-derived, yeast-fermented alcoholic beverages, cigarette smoke, chemically synthesized drugs and narcotics are. I am sure you have heard people call themselves "chocaholics," "cake-aholics," or "junk-foodaholics." They do it not realizing how true it really is.

I, Fran, remember having lunch with David Kirsh, "The No-Cal King." We were talking about the different flavorings he used in his No-Cal sodas, and with much pride he went into the other room and brought in a bottle of his brand-new No-Cal chocolate soda, not yet introduced to the public. He said he'd had to develop the chocolate flavor because he himself was a chocaholic and suspected that most other people were, too. Chocaholic—addicted to chocolate.

I believe that many of us who love chocolate would good-naturedly agree that we are chocaholics and could easily binge on it given the chance, knowing full well it will, among other things, cause us to gain weight. But what about those of us who love bread or popcorn or cottage cheese or potatoes with gravy and make one of these a mainstay of our diets, eating it day after day, meal after meal? Could we be addicted to wheat (bread), corn, milk, or potato?

The answer is an emphatic *yes*. Yes, we could, and many of us are overweight and miserable because we are eating compulsively as a result of these very common and extremely important food addictions.

When Marshall was on his last book tour for *Dr. Mandell's 5-Day*

Allergy Relief System, he stopped at a diner to have lunch. The menu amazed him. As he opened it, there was a large page for "Specials of the Day." One-quarter of the page, in big black letters surrounded by a box, said, TUESDAY SPECIAL: BISCUITS AND GRAVY. He knew from some of his wheat-addicted patients that they could and did make a meal out of wheat biscuits and wheat-laden gravy, but he'd never expected to see it listed as a special in a restaurant! Just across the aisle from him was a woman with triple chins, balloon arms, and an enormous abdomen, who was having trouble getting into her seat. She announced to the waiter, "I don't need a menu. I came for the Tuesday Special." Well, folks, you now understand what that meal order was all about.

Watching with horrified fascination as she cleaned her plate, Marshall couldn't help thinking that he was viewing a tragedy and that he should tell this victim of food addiction what was really happening to her.

As with all addictions, if you don't "feed" them constantly, you suffer withdrawal symptoms. Withdrawal symptoms are our "self-inflicted punishment" for not giving our addicted bodies what they demand. They come in many uncomfortable forms, and most people are probably familiar with them as the aches and pains of everyday living. Marshall has repeatedly shown that joint pain, exhaustion, depression, unexplained anger, restlessness, headaches, dizziness, indigestion, constipation, and many other maladies of life are in many cases the withdrawal symptoms of a food-addicted person who may have been misdiagnosed as a case of psychosomatic illness. So it is not surprising that compulsive eating is a reaction to the cravings caused by the conscious and unconscious need to prevent or relieve the uncomfortable withdrawal symptoms of food addiction.

People who fail on other diets are a good example of addiction to frequently eaten foods. When patients who have been on Weight Watchers come to the Center, Marshall knows almost without seeing them that they are probably having problems with the foods they have been eating most often—fruits and vegetables, including grapefruit, celery, lettuce, broccoli, etc.; fish; chicken; and eggs. He also knows that he must test these people for chemical sensitivity, especially to the coal-tar-derived chemicals (like the sweeteners, synthetic coloring agents, and artificial flavors found in diet foods and sodas).

Sue Horn, a patient at the Center who tried the Weight Watchers Diet as an adolescent, not only couldn't stick to the diet but wound up so depressed that she consulted a psychiatrist. She now understands why. Sue is sensitive to some of the chemically derived coloring, flavoring, and/or preservatives in diet drinks. When she drank diet soda or ate foods with artificial sweeteners, she immediately became extremely depressed and bloated.

When Sue was on the Weight Watchers Diet, which allowed her diet soda and tea with saccharin, her depression led her to feel "Nobody cares about me—what does it matter what I look like?" And this was compounded by severe hunger; so off she went on an eating binge that, even to her, looked like an emotional reaction. She did not realize that her appetite was terribly overstimulated because of an allergic response to the saccharin.

By the time she came home from school in the afternoon, she'd be feeling tired and depressed from drinking diet soda or tea with artificial sweeteners. To cheer herself up, she would bake sugary cookies, rationalizing that she was just making them "for the family." She knew her family loved chocolate chip cookies, but she would end up eating so many, there would be hardly any left for anyone else.

Through Marshall's testing, Sue has learned that she has an allergy-like sensitivity to chemicals and that this includes fruit tree sprays. Whenever she eats commercially raised fresh fruit containing spray residues, she begins to crave all things sweet. Just about the same time Sue went to Weight Watchers, she took a four-week trip to Europe. Four weeks of vacationing and eating anything and everything she wanted. During that time Sue lost 25 pounds despite daily pasta in Italy, wine, and gourmet meals in restaurants. She couldn't believe it. She felt and looked terrific. Her family was thrilled.

Hoping to keep her weight down when she came home, Sue was extremely careful about what she ate. Yet after just a few weeks of "dieting," she had gained back all of her weight and was very depressed. Now she knows that it was a result of the pesticide residues, preservatives, and artificial sweeteners she was eating, and had consumed much less of while eating better-quality food in Europe. But she didn't know it then. Sue's psychiatrist interpreted her depression as something wrong in her home life; she began to believe that her problem was psychological, and she felt very ashamed. Sue could never talk to anyone about it—not even her family. It wasn't until years later that a friend told her about Marshall. Sue has been on our rotation diet for well over a year and after losing 15 pounds is a slim size 12. She now weighs 138 and at 5'7" she looks great. Best of all, she has found, "I'm really a happy person!"

ADDICTIVE FOOD ALLERGY

As we have said, addictive food allergy is a condition similar to compulsive drinking, narcotic addiction, or compulsive cigarette smoking. When we eat a food over and over again, possibly several times a day, day after day, our bodies can become biologically dependent upon (addicted to) that food and crave it. If we do not answer this biologic need by eating the food, we will experience physical and/or mental withdrawal symptoms in much the same way compulsive smokers would if they could not light up and inhale the chemicals in a cigarette. Alcoholics and drug addicts have a similar problem. The withdrawal symptoms occur within a certain number of hours (the exact amount of time varies from person to person and from food to food) after we have eaten an addictive food.

The ways to relieve withdrawal symptoms are to try to completely or partially block the symptoms with medication, or do what most addicts do—eat the addicting food again. For example, if your withdrawal period for a particular food is ten hours and you ate a food you were addicted to for dinner at 6:00 P.M., your withdrawal symptoms would start around 4:00 A.M., probably waking you up with monotonous regularity. The symptoms could take almost any form, including itching, headache, rapid pulse, joint pain (arthritis), respiratory problems (nasal obstruction, asthma), digestive-tract symptoms, depression, anxiety, insomnia, and even nightmares. These symptoms might persist for hours or could be relieved by eating the food or foods from dinner that produced these addictive withdrawal symptoms. Some people have become accustomed to keeping a convenient form of their addictive food on their night tables and just reach out and eat it when they awaken, without even getting out of bed.

In chronic, addictive food allergy, the delayed symptoms of food withdrawal may occur three or four hours after a meal, or they may not appear for eight to twelve hours or longer. The withdrawal symptoms will be relieved by eating the addictive food—or they will gradually clear in three or four days if the food is eliminated from the diet.

Someone addicted to wheat could begin the day with a doughnut, toast, pancakes, Danish, Wheaties, or a Pop-Tart for breakfast; followed by soup with crackers, a sandwich and pie for lunch; and rolls, spaghetti, and cake at dinner. It is possible that a person with this addiction would find cookies and milk a most pleasant bedtime snack, thereby completing a day's addictive cycle.

One of our wheat-addicted patients, Andrew Alexander, Sr., today a successful computer technician, came to the Center weighing 35 pounds over his desired weight. He had not always been heavy. Andrew put the weight on after a knee injury that kept him out of work for a year and a half. He had worked for the electric light company, reading meters, a job that kept him active and on his feet. He walked nine miles a day. After sitting around and eating all day, he found himself becoming progressively more obese and he did not like it. He tried to diet, but the weight would not move.

When he came to the Center, he had many allergy problems, including a chronic and very annoying sinus condition associated with frequent sore throats.

As Marshall reviewed Andrew's eating habits, he immediately recognized where his overweight problem came from. He said he went to bed early but got up regularly at midnight and had to go out to get a burrito or pizza. He would actually get out of bed and go to his local 7-Eleven store to get a burrito! While he was there, he would pick up some coffee cake and doughnuts for breakfast "with all of the sugary marshmallows and goos. I'd always start out the day with my pastries." For lunch, Andrew had a hamburger on a bun or a tuna sandwich on rye bread. Upon coming home from work, he'd have a toasted cheese sandwich, batter-fried chicken, hot rolls, or chicken with dumplings—only to awaken again every midnight craving his burrito or pizza.

We asked Andrew if he had any idea why he was eating this way. "No, just that I was hungry, and I had to have something, so that's what I did." We asked him what happened when he tried to diet and not eat these foods. He answered emphatically, "The Hungry Horrors!" He felt hungry soon after each meal, no matter how much he had eaten. He felt he had to have a snack, craving a peanut butter and jelly sandwich.

It seemed impossible to Andrew, at that time, to give up his much-beloved wheat. But he did. He went on a diet like the one in this book, broke his wheat addiction within a few days, and lost those 35 pounds of unwanted fat and allergically retained water without taking any diuretics or drugs. Many of his chronic illnesses and aches and pains went, too, including that series of very uncomfortable sore throats he had had for eight years!

There are millions of individuals who, like Sue and Andrew, have addictive allergies and don't even know it. And in most cases, these allergies are causing their overweight and many other health problems.

MASKED FOOD ALLERGY

Have you ever gone on a diet and felt irritable? Did you think your irritability came from having too little to eat? Well, that might have been so, but chances are the reason was that you were having a mild allergic brain reaction that was a withdrawal symptom of food addiction. You were not eating your favorite foods—those withdrawal-blocking addictive foods you eat every day, love and depend upon for comfort and a general feeling of well-being. You may not know what they are now because you probably have just eaten them and are comfortable. Unless they have been identified for you, you don't know what your masked food allergies are. We eat these allergically addictive foods so often that we really do not know what it feels like to be without them. Our allergy is "masked"—covered over.

If a fasting day is part of your religion, this scene may be familiar to you. In the Jewish religion our fasting day is Yom Kippur, a day spent at religious services. By the end of the day, many of the congregation are fidgeting, restless, headachy, and cranky. We watch people who have spent hours without their favorite addictive foods slowly going into food withdrawal, shifting in their chairs as they anxiously await sundown. And we believe that if we could read their minds about four or five o'clock in the afternoon, we would know exactly what foods they were planning to eat to break their fast.

Marshall has a research fantasy in which he goes to the synagogue to meet the congregation just as services are breaking for the day. Everyone is ready to go home and eat, but he stands in the doorway and asks each person how they feel and exactly what they are going to eat—a piece of cheese, a glass of milk, orange juice, coffee, a hard-boiled egg, or a big slab of rye bread with butter. He knows that they know exactly what they are going to eat, and he knows that whatever the food is, there is an excellent chance that it will make them feel better. But instead of allowing the congregation to go home and eat, Marshall would take them to a lavishly prepared feast replete with every food except the ones they were craving.

I told you it was an allergist's fantasy, but the results of it would be very real. There almost certainly would be a room filled with people eating great amounts of food, but not satisfying their hunger or able to rid themselves of their physical and mental discomfort. They would have a living introduction to what addictive food allergy really is and how it can cause compulsive eating.

IT'S NOT YOUR FAULT YOU'RE FAT

We hope you are getting the idea that we weren't kidding when we named our book *It's Not Your Fault You're Fat*. And we hope that at this very minute you will put all of those painful years of blaming yourself for your eating binges behind you and join us on the road to slimness and good health. In the next pages, we will kick our allergies and addictions, rid ourselves of the excess body fluids and fat caused by them, and emerge the beautiful, healthy people we all are. We know you can do it—it's easy.

2

THE WEIGHTY PROBLEM
OF WATER RETENTION

Many patients who come to the Alan Mandell Center tell Marshall that they can gain or lose large amounts of weight overnight—often 3 to 5 pounds or more. Andrea Camps is one of these people. Andrea gained a surprising 11 pounds overnight, although her total intake of food for the day had been less than 9 ounces. It included:

1 wheat cracker
1 teaspoon caviar
4 ounces filet mignon
7 green beans
4 mushrooms
½ ounce Brie cheese
⅛ of an apple

Andrea was frustrated and upset. She had not been faithful to the diet we had prescribed for her, but she had eaten so little food! What could have happened?

What could have happened—and did—was that Andrea had an allergic reaction to a food or foods she had eaten, and her allergic symptom was water retention.

Marshall has found that water retention can be responsible for 5 to 10 pounds or more of excess body weight (one patient characteristically retained and lost 25 pounds of fluid). You may not know if you are carrying a few or many pounds of excess water. The fluid retained in your body can be so evenly distributed, you may not be aware that you are waterlogged. Of course, if you have clearly visible puffiness of the eyes, face, or lips, or swelling of the hands, feet, or ankles, you will know.

Whenever I spend a day in New York City, my hands swell to the point of having to remove my rings, and I get large dark swellings under my eyes that Marshall and other allergists refer to as "allergic shiners." When I lived in New York, I had these dark swellings to some degree all the time, but dismissed them as a product of aging. Many of my friends had facial puffiness and similar eye swellings and were given "water pills" (diuretics) to get rid of the puffiness.

These "bags under the eyes" are localized areas of "allergic edema." Allergic edema, or water retention, is one of the most misunderstood problems of overweight. It is a reversible disorder of the capillaries, those delicate, thin-walled blood vessels that carry nourishment to all parts of the body. During an allergic reaction, some of the fluid that is part of the blood plasma leaks through the allergically enlarged pores of the temporarily malfunctioning capillaries into the surrounding tissue, causing it to puff up with fluid. We call this condition "edema."

When the food or chemical that caused the allergic reaction is no longer present in the body, the walls of the capillaries return to normal and stop leaking fluid. The "allergic" fluid that has leaked into the tissues returns to the general circulation and is eliminated by the kidneys, excreted through the skin, or evaporated through the lungs, taking with it important *pounds* of your unnecessary water weight in the form of allergic-edema fluid—and leaving a thinner, healthier you.

There are varying degrees of edema. One type that everybody has experienced is the mosquito bite. The female mosquito injects saliva in order to keep the blood from coagulating so that she can get a nice long free meal from the person she has bitten. The body reacts to the mosquito's saliva by causing the capillary blood vessels at the site of the bite to dilate and leak a small amount of watery blood plasma into the surrounding tissues. The temporary bump that appears in the skin results from the capillary damage that only affects a small area. But a person who is extremely sensitive and highly allergic to something in mosquito saliva will get a huge reaction in the form of a giant bite that may be two or more inches in diameter. In many instances, the local injury may not be reversible and there may be local tissue breakdown that heals very slowly with the formation of a persistent scab and loss of skin pigment.

Hives are another form of edema. Small hives often look exactly like a crop of small mosquito bites. Larger hives can resemble pancakes piled on top of each other with their edges overlapping. Giant hives are large, generalized areas of swelling that at times may look like a deformity. They are the puffy areas seen on and above the lips or under and over the eyes. Sometimes the eyes are almost completely closed. When the cheeks are also involved, the person takes on a porky appearance.

Hives and other localized allergic swellings can occur in any part of the body, not just the skin. They have even been known to form on the outer surface of the brain—an observation made by a neurosurgeon during brain surgery. When an area of the brain swells, its function may be seriously altered for as long as the allergic reaction lasts. This interference with normal brain function may cause inability to concentrate, depression, headache, confusion, nervousness, fatigue, irritability, unprovoked anger, poor memory, behavioral changes, difficulty with perception, learning problems, mood swings, and even schizophrenia.

Dr. Bernard S. Zussman of Memphis, Tennessee, had an allergic patient with a surgical opening in his skull from an earlier operation, and his observation of this man supports the conclusion that brain swellings may cause many important symptoms in the nervous system. Dr. Zussman's patient's brain would swell and even expand slightly out of the "surgical hole," pushing up on his overlying scalp whenever he ate something that he was "brain-allergic" to.

So next time you have a headache or are experiencing one of the symptoms mentioned above and feel you need a favorite food to stop the feeling, think of Dr. Zussman's patient and don't eat. Tell yourself that you need a swollen brain and all the unwanted symptoms of brain allergy like you need a hole in your head!

DIURETICS

One way to rid yourself of excess water is to take a diuretic—a "water pill." Diuretics are drugs that cause the kidneys to eliminate water, but unfortunately, the fluid that is removed is rapidly replaced; therefore, "water pills" must be taken on a continuing basis or they are ineffective. *Diuretics do not eliminate the cause of the fluid retention*—they only temporarily remove some of the fluid.

There are many types of diuretics, and, like most other drugs, they may cause side effects in some people, the most important being the removal of too much of some minerals from the body, especially potassium, which can be lost along with the (retained) water that is being excreted. Without adequate potassium, we can experience weakness and fatigue—but that's not all. A heavy loss of potassium, although unlikely, could have a negative effect on the heart, blood, kidneys, muscles, nerves, and skin. Acne could develop; you might be thirsty all the time; your skin might get dry; you could become constipated, nervous, unable to sleep, suffer muscle spasms, and experience a slow, irregular heartbeat. It has also been reported that diuretics impair male sexual function (both drive and performance)! It hardly seems worth taking the chance.

On our diet, we can almost guarantee that you will not need diuretics if there is no other medical reason for you to take them. The It's Not Your Fault You're Fat Diet removes or controls the dietary causes of your allergic edema, thereby "eliminating" it from your life. No more swollen hands and ankles, puffy faces, and distended tummies. They will be a part of yesterday.

The Honorable John Barritt, Bermuda's Speaker of the House, is a patient at the Center. He came to us with ringing in his ears, eye irritation, and an occasionally protruding, bloated abdomen. He was given an individualized rotation diet that was based on the results of food allergy tests. Within a few weeks, his eye and ear symptoms came under control and he lost 20 pounds. He told us that he had always watched his weight, but his abdominal distention had never disappeared permanently until this diet: "My stomach would protrude and recede, protrude and recede."

Now John feels that he may possibly be a little bit underweight and he is coming back to the Center, where we can observe him for a while to determine if he should gain a few pounds. Too much of a good thing! (But Marshall thinks John may have achieved his truly normal weight level and may have to get used to his new trim appearance. We should all have to face this problem!)

John Barritt's abdominal problem was a combination of intestinal distension due to food allergy and allergic fluid retention, localized edema. He could always see when he was becoming distended, but, as we have told you, this is not always the case; edema is often spread so evenly over the body that you may not know you have allergic water retention. If you are a person with this generalized type of hidden water retention and have had problems losing weight on other diets, you will be most pleasantly surprised to see how your waterlogged pounds will quickly disappear on our diet.

Mary Raush is in her sixties. She and her husband live in Middletown, New Jersey. Mary came to see Marshall because she had a persistent cough that was getting progressively worse. She had been to other allergists, taken shots, and gotten no results. At the time she came to the Center, Mary did not think she was overweight. She was 5'1" and weighed 120 pounds. Marshall tested her and found her to be allergic to many foods. His treatment for her allergies included placing her on a Rotary Diversified Diet, like the one you will find in Chapter 9. In two months, Mary found that she was 22 pounds lighter after eliminating the edema fluid. She went on a maintenance diet and has now stabilized at 100 pounds—her proper weight. She now feels very comfortable with her weight and realizes that she was overweight and did not know it.

As you can see, allergic edema is a very important culprit in overweight. By ridding ourselves of our allergically retained excess water, we can become slimmer and healthier. This diet can do that for you.

You may be asking yourself what will happen if you haven't any allergies that you are aware of. Will this diet work for you if you haven't any water to lose?

If you are overweight, it is not very likely that you are free of food addiction or without some excess water weight. Physicians like Marshall see very few cases of overweight people who are not allergic or who do not have some degree of obvious or hidden edema. If you have ever gone on a diet and lost more than 3½ pounds the first week, you were losing excess water. On a complete water fast with no foods whatsoever, it is only possible to lose (or metabolize) a maximum of 3½ pounds of fat a week.

IF I HAVE ALLERGIC EDEMA, HOW DID I GET IT?

Any food that you are sensitive to can cause allergic edema. As we discussed in chapter 1, it is believed that most sensitivities to foods develop from eating them too often. It is possible to be allergic to a substance without having obvious edema from it, as each allergic reaction brings with it a unique set of symptoms. However, the basic allergic reaction does involve capillary leakage most of the time. Some allergies cause joint pain, some cause digestive problems, still others cause respiratory disorders or other problems, but *the allergic reactions that cause you to gain weight are those that trigger compulsive eating and/or those that cause allergic edema.*

Susan Wilmington is a writer and a patient at our Center. As a child, Susan was underweight—her classmates called her "skinny bones." Her weight remained low until she became pregnant, when she gained 45 pounds. That is when her addictive food allergies started to become severe. She was hungry all the time. Right after her son was born, while she was still in the hospital, she broke out in hives and a generalized flushing of the skin. The allergic skin reaction was so bad that she looked as if she had been burned. The doctors thought it might have happened because of her exposure to the many bouquets of flowers in her room. From then on, she suffered terribly with allergies.

When Susan came to Marshall and was tested, she was found to be allergic to many substances, including over 90% of the foods she was tested for. But only three of all of these offending foods caused her to suddenly gain weight. Wheat, yeast, and cane sugar produced acute allergic reactions in her capillaries, causing her to gain 5 pounds overnight each time she ate one of those foods. Susan knows now that her rapid 5-pound weight gains are not 5 pounds of fat. They are 5 pounds of water and can be easily lost by going back on her allergen-free diet.

As you look through the diets in chapters 8 and 9, you will find that they include almost every food you have ever eaten and many that you may never have tried. There undoubtedly will be some foods listed that you are allergically sensitive to, and it is very likely that you will have reactions to them, so if you mysteriously gain a pound or two overnight, don't be upset; chances are the excess weight will be gone within a day or two in addition to the weight loss of that day. On our diet, we want you to weigh yourself daily. We want you to know right away if you have eaten a food or foods that cause you to gain weight, so you can promptly take them out of your diet for a month or longer until you regain tolerance for them.

When I first went on the It's Not Your Fault You're Fat Diet, I immediately learned that I had problems of weight gain on my bread day. The fourteenth day of the diet, we eat bread and butter, with spaghetti and butter sauce for lunch. Thank heaven I was too full to get to the spaghetti, because the bread alone caused me to gain 4 pounds. I was so happy I knew about allergic edema. The 4 pounds were gone by the following morning and so was 1 pound more.

ALLERGIC EDEMA AND CHEMICALS

Allergic edema can result not only from a sensitivity to foods but also from a wide variety of chemical substances we eat, drink, or breathe. Some people actually gain weight on diet foods. If you have been dieting and dieting and you know you are sticking to it even though nobody else believes you, the reason you have not been losing weight could well be the diet soda you are drinking or the prepared diet foods you are eating. The artificial sweeteners, flavors, coloring agents, preservatives, and other additives in these products could be causing you to retain fluids.

Sandra Kierz has an interesting story to tell. Sandra grew up on Long Island. Her mother and grandmother kept wonderful vegetable gardens and each year they froze and canned the foods to eat all year long. So Sandra grew up on Long Island fish and homegrown vegetables.

When Sandra married, she moved to Milwaukee. Her husband is Polish and loved sausage, ham, salami, and other prepared meats. She started cooking these foods for him, and of course she ate them, too. She began to gain weight without wanting to. Before she knew it, she weighed 170 pounds. Sandra decided to diet: She ate salads with low-calorie dressings, she cut back on eating starches like potatoes and rice, and got to the point where everything she ate was diet food—diet mayonnaise, diet margarine, diet soda, diet bread. And she kept gaining weight.

Sandra thought, "Well, you hit a certain age and you automatically gain weight." But she was only 25! What's more, she and her husband own a general store. She runs around all day long in the store and gets plenty of exercise. They open the store at seven in the morning and don't leave until ten at night.

Sandra's mother gave her a copy of Marshall's first allergy-relief book, and as soon as she read what he had written about chemicals, she immediately decided to cut them out of her diet. She realized that in order to avoid consuming calories, she had gone on an all-chemical diet.

Today Sandra says she eats all of those "high-calorie" foods she'd been avoiding and has lost all of her excess weight. (She went from 175 pounds to 130 pounds and is able to eat three times the amount she used to.) By just going off the chemicals associated with diet foods, Sandra lost 20 pounds in three weeks. "It just came off," she says. Unbelievable? We don't think so. We have seen it happen to quite a few other happier and healthier patients.

DRUGS MAY CAUSE WATER RETENTION

Another phenomenon we see that is always very distressing to patients is water retention caused by medication.

Steroids that suppress allergies and inflammation are the most common drugs that cause edema. Cortisone derivatives like prednisone, prednisolone, medrol, and other steroids are used to treat many conditions, including arthritis, asthma, and colitis. Steroids are potent drugs, and physicians treat them with great respect, recognizing their many potential serious side effects, one of which is fluid retention.

Maxine Rolnick, a physical therapist, came to see Marshall because she had suddenly developed asthma and her doctors could not find the cause of it. She also had severe fatigue and a weight problem.

Maxine's weight problem had begun after she had a hysterectomy (Marshall suspects that a chemical overload of anesthetics started it all). She gained 10 pounds that she could not lose. Allergic bronchial asthma became an added problem, for which she was given cortisone, and soon thereafter she began to balloon. She felt that she couldn't get rid of her excess pounds, and then she came to the Alan Mandell Center.

When Maxine was given comprehensive antiallergy treatment, including our rotation diet, she lost 30 pounds, her asthma improved, her fatigue disappeared, and she felt much better overall. The steroid-caused edema and the allergic fluid retention were both controlled by nondrug medical management. Many of her problems disappeared, including a serious problem with high blood pressure. At 54 years of age, she is able to work full-time as a physical therapist, a most demanding job.

Erica Johnson, a 40-year-old housewife from Oregon, had been given prednisone for her allergic, rheumatoid arthritis. She "blew up" so much from this steroid that she stopped going out of the house—she hated people's "pregnant" jokes. She came to Marshall for a total evaluation of her problems and went on our diet. Most of her arthritis has cleared and she has lost the edema she suffered as a side effect of the drug. She also lost the allergic edema associated with her very severe arthritis.

Jane Misuraca gained weight following an infectious illness treated with antibiotics for a year. She had a fever all the time and did not feel hungry, but "All of a sudden I just started puffing up. I gained thirty-five pounds." Marshall believes that the long-term stress of this infection initiated or triggered potential allergies.

About twenty months ago, Jane came to the Center. She was tested, treated, and put on a rotary diet. In six weeks she lost 30 pounds. "It just melted off." When she came back to the Center for a checkup, her allergic facial edema had cleared up and nobody on the staff recognized her because we had never seen her normal nonpuffy face.

EDEMA AND THE SALT CONTROVERSY

We allow you to have salt on our diet. Many of our recipes say "sea salt to taste." If your kidneys are functioning properly, your body will probably excrete 98% of the salt you take in during the day. You need some salt to keep your mineral balance right.

Some of our patients appear to be sensitive to some forms of salt but not others. Sandra Boogertman finds sea salt is fine, but baking powder and baking soda cause her to bloat. Table salt may contain corn-derived glucose that can affect some people. You will have to experiment for yourself. If you seem to retain water from salt, you can try Morton Lite Salt (or another salt substitute you can tolerate) to see if that makes a difference.

Now you know that the It's Not Your Fault You're Fat Diet can do two things for you: (1) It will help you to find out which foods you are consciously or unknowingly eating compulsively—and how to remove them from your diet; (2) it will help you to identify which foods may be causing your allergic edema—and remove them from your diet.

You will find as thousands have before you that it works. Read on to learn about its principles.

3

DR. MANDELL DISCUSSES THE ALLERGY-OVERWEIGHT CONNECTION

ARE YOU ALLERGIC?

Any overweight individual is likely to be allergic or in some way sensitive—reactive—to several or many of the substances he or she comes in contact with during normal daily activities. Just being alive and carrying out the essential life-sustaining functions of eating, drinking, and breathing in our synthetic-filled and chemically polluted environment can be enough to initiate, aggravate, and perpetuate an overweight condition, along with many other ailments. Medically significant overweight affects one out of six Americans—more than 40 million out of a population of over 230 million. This condition is often associated with a wide variety of major and minor physical ailments. It also can produce "psychiatric" disorders that in many instances are of allergic or bio-ecologic origin.

To show you just how widespread allergic disorders are, here are some important facts to consider. According to Dr. Howard G. Rapaport, a conventional allergist, the common allergies like hay fever, hives, eczema, and asthma affect half the American population. The U.S. Department of Commerce has reported that, in a single year, more than $50 million was spent on antihistamines, more than $100 million was spent on injections of patients by conventional allergists and chest specialists, and $170 million worth of drugs were purchased to dilate congested and constricted bronchial tubes.

ALLERGIC REACTIONS ARE OFTEN MISDIAGNOSED

Many environmentally ill people, suffering from complex disorders characterized by frustrating, misinterpreted combinations of symptoms that perplex their many consultants, have become medical dropouts. And great numbers of their misdiagnosed fellow sufferers have been consigned to the psychiatric or psychological category—an enormous, overworked, and most convenient medical wastebasket. There is also an abundance of very respectable multiple-symptom disorders that are usually assumed, but rarely confirmed, to be the result of an invasion by some nasty little viruses.

The 1980 *World Almanac and Book of Facts* reports that there were over 400,000 admissions to mental hospitals in 1975 and over 6 million "patient care episodes" in which people consulted with doctors about psychological or psychiatric problems. One government official states that over 20 million people in this country (10% of the American public) are in urgent need of psychological or psychiatric care. My colleagues and I are convinced by our clinical experience that an overwhelming majority of these cases of so-called mental illness are allergic/bio-ecologic disorders of the nervous system associated with various reversible malfunctions in other organs and systems.[1]

Depression has been referred to as "the common cold of mental disturbances." We find it also ranks high among the prominent and frequently occurring allergic or allergylike bio-ecologic disorders of the brain. Not all cases of hard-to-explain depression are of bio-ecologic causation, but many are. This is not to deny that those sad life experiences that everyone compassionately recognizes as understandable causes of great unhappiness—such as the death of a loved one, losing one's job, a divorce, etc.—may sometimes precipitate a state of depression. Some depressions are responses to severe psychological stress, but emotionally precipitated depression is less frequent than most people, including psychiatrists, realize.

Depression is often misdiagnosed as the underlying "cause" of many physical and mental symptoms. One of my allergic patients who suffered from severe migraine headaches for many years was informed by her

[1] I conceived the terms "bio-ecologic mental illness" and "bio-ecologic diseases" in 1972 to emphasize the importance of biologic factors (such as heredity, physiology, biochemistry, metabolism, and nutrition) in each person's degree of susceptibility to environmental factors. It is because of varying degrees of deficiencies or malfunctions in these biologic and biochemical areas that a person is more or less vulnerable to the effects of ecologic factors in the food, water, and air required for human existence. In order to have an illness, one must be biologically capable of developing that disorder after being exposed to its environmental cause(s).

This concept was introduced to the scientific world in a paper I presented on bio-ecologic mental illness at the First World Congress of Biologic Psychiatry, held in Buenos Aires in 1973. Since that time, many colleagues have adopted the term "bio-ecologic," and it is being used more and more in medical literature. There now are organizations and a medical foundation that have—to my great satisfaction—used my term to identify themselves. About fifteen years ago, I coined the terms "allergic addiction," "addictive allergy," and "allergylike sensitivities," which have also become part of the scientific and popular literature.

psychiatrist that her chronic head pains were due to the mysterious work-
ings of her unconscious mind. He said that she had "a fantastic ability to
punish herself with these headaches," and went on to explain that she was
depressed "because of unconscious guilt feelings," and that because of
some unspecified guilt-generating action in the past, she made herself
suffer frequent episodes of severe head pain associated with nausea and
vomiting.

The psychiatric diagnosis in this case was 100% wrong. When I reviewed this patient's dietary exposures, she gave me the diagnostic clue
that led to our acquitting her wrongly accused subconscious mind as the
impartial dispenser of justice and punishment. I learned that she was
drinking one to two pots of coffee every day—a daily intake of eight to
sixteen cups of coffee. And guess what happened when I took her to the
laboratory and tested her by placing under her tongue a few drops of an
allergenic extract prepared from coffee? Less than five minutes after the
test was given, she was slowly rocking back and forth in her chair, holding
her throbbing head between her hands. A few drops of coffee extract had
duplicated her chronic, agonizing symptoms.

In those few minutes, she was convinced that her unconscious mind
was not on a self-punishing "guilt trip." The headache was relieved by a
symptom-neutralizing dose of highly diluted coffee extract, her guilt was
banished, and I "cured" her "emotional disorder" by suggesting that she
stop drinking her favorite beverage. Her subsequent freedom from migraine attacks confirmed my diagnosis of recurrent headaches due to food
allergy.

The diagnosis of "unconscious guilt" by her honest and sincere,
board-certified psychiatrist was only mere speculation. His professional
competence was seriously limited because his training did not give him
even an elementary working knowledge of bio-ecologic disorders of the
nervous system.

There is evidence that bio-ecologic mental illness affects 50–75% or
more of psychiatric patients. Depression is responsible for about 2 million
suicide attempts each year, in which about 30,000 of our unfortunate fellow humans succeed.

Twenty million Americans suffering from the violent mood swings
of manic-depressive illness were reported in 1976. Many cases of this
"psychotic" condition—the big brother of what is known to pediatricians
as the allergic tension-fatigue disorder of childhood—are of bio-ecologic
origin. In 1974, there were 2 million reported cases of schizophrenia in
this country. My colleagues in orthomolecular psychiatry and clinical
ecology are certain that at least 75% and perhaps many more of these
individuals suffer from a reversible allergylike disorder associated with

partially understood biochemical abnormalities and unmet needs for specific vitamins, minerals, and amino acids.

Many headaches are the result of unsuspected allergic reactions. In 1964, almost 25 million people sought medical assistance for this condition. Headaches affect one out of every eight people in this country, and in 1977 we spent over $500 million on pain relievers and aspirin.

Allergic fatigue, too, affects huge numbers of people, many of whom awaken each morning to face an energyless day of greatly decreased productivity. These allergy sufferers are more tired in the morning than they were when they went to bed for a night of unrefreshing sleep. In 1979, *U.S. News & World Report* published an article in which a Pennsylvania physician estimated that one-half of the hospitalized patients in this country reported fatigue as one of their major health problems.

The preceding information gives you a partial overview of our current medical situation and indicates the frequency and importance of some of the common symptomatically treated disorders—often allergic in nature—that affect great numbers of people, including many overweight individuals. Some other disorders that also belong to this group include arthritis, colitis, "indigestion," constipation, urinary-tract disorders, repeated episodes of flulike illness, itching, "nervousness," restlessness, dizziness, blurred vision, anxiety, irritability, insomnia, short attention span, learning and reading difficulties, confusion, poor memory, impaired concentration, and many other physical and mental ailments.

In brief, we live in a poorly nourished, carelessly and dangerously polluted industrial civilization. Its citizens suffer from numerous allergic and allergylike bio-ecologic diseases of body and "mind" that are filling our hospitals, clinics, and the offices of members of the healing profession. Allergic-addictive overweight is an important facet of this widespread group of serious health problems.

HOW ARE THE ALLERGIES THAT CAUSE OVERWEIGHT DIAGNOSED AND TREATED?

In diagnosis of allergic-addictive overweight and the identification of its usually multiple causes, a well-informed patient is his or her own best friend and an invaluable asset to the physician. In my practice, it is my policy to have each new patient read my book on internal allergies[2]

---

[2] Marshall Mandell, M.D., and Lynn Waller Scanlon, *Dr. Mandell's 5-Day Allergy Relief System* (New York: Pocket Books, 1980).

before coming to Norwalk for their initial consultation. Almost every patient finds information and case histories that relate to his or her problem, and the book often describes some aspects of their illness so closely that it is not unusual for the new patient to identify with the people they read about.

Patient History

I also ask all patients to prepare for our initial consultation by writing a short or long (as the case requires) chronologic health history, in their own words. This history provides invaluable observations that permit me to follow the development of the usually multiple-symptom, multiple-system complaints that they suffered from in the past as well as currently active ones. I also request that they include information concerning the places where they have lived, and their exposures to potential sources of illness in their work environment and at home, including their hobby area.

I want to know the effects of foods and alcoholic beverages, what happens to them when meals are missed, what their condition is after eating binges, and exactly how they feel "the morning after." I ask them to report on any matter they think may be important to any aspect of their physical and mental health. This certainly includes comments about anything they may have learned about themselves as they read my book.

You, the patient, are always there when the reaction-inducing exposures occur and when the resulting symptoms appear. You are the deeply concerned, on-the-scene expert regarding all of the circumstances related to your bio-ecologic disorder. At this time, you may or may not completely understand the basic nature of your problem and it is possible that your interpretation of the specific facts concerning it may not be entirely correct. However, your observations and those of other individuals who know you well contain fundamental data that often are of great diagnostic value. In almost every instance, such observations are loaded with highly suggestive diagnostic clues.

Further information is obtained from the comprehensive questionnaire that each patient completes before his or her consultation. One section concerns symptoms affecting each body system, and the more check marks I find, the more likely it is that the patient has a bio-ecologic illness. The questionnaire provides detailed information about all of the patient's exposures and reactions to environmental factors, foods, alcoholic beverages, drugs, chemical fumes (pollution), and airborne allergens. The questionnaire is also constructed to double-check certain important areas by seeking the same information by means of differently worded questions. In almost every case, important information is obtained that directs my attention to various almost-certain or highly likely factors that play a major role in the patient's illness. (You will have the opportunity to fill out similar questionnaires in chapter 5.)

On many occasions, as I carefully reviewed the information in a patient's chronologically arranged notes and questionnaire, searching for cause-and-effect relationships between exposures and symptoms, the pieces of their puzzling and misdiagnosed long-term chronic misery fell into place. The facts of the case described in a patient's notes were "waving red flags at me" directing my attention to additional areas to be discussed during our consultation and to be investigated during the testing that follows our evaluation of each patient's history.

At the conclusion of a consultation, it is frequently evident to the new patient that he or she has a number of allergies or allergylike sensitivities and/or addictions. Our remaining problem is to identify the specific causes of particular symptoms.

Food addiction is the most common form of food allergy. This diet-related disorder causes compulsive eating, compulsive drinking, and many kinds of middle-of-the-night ailments, and is responsible for premeal or missed-meal withdrawal symptoms (often mistaken for hypoglycemia). Food addiction is usually very easy to diagnose once it is suspected. Chemical sensitivities often stand out like the unmistakable evidence of a recent skunk spraying. (By the time you finish reading the interpretations of your questionnaire answers in Chapter 5, you will see exactly what I mean.)

Skin Tests Don't Work in Food and Chemical Allergy

Conventional skin testing is of very little value (80% error) in diagnosing food allergy, useless in most cases of sensitivity to environmental chemicals (in food, water, and air), and only fairly accurate in the identification of airborne allergens like dusts, animal danders, molds, and pollens. I discontinued this method of testing twenty years ago in favor of the much more accurate and information-loaded symptom-duplicating techniques known as "provocative testing."

I am not going to waste your valuable reading time, or space in this volume, to review the food industry–backed and emotionally charged resistance to provocative testing by physicians who have closed their minds to this well proven diagnostic method. It is sufficient to assure you that you need *pay absolutely no attention to anyone who "does not believe in food allergy" as a major cause of common and often serious bodywide disorders.* I only ask that you give yourself a golden opportunity to lose weight and become healthier by controlling your hidden and addictive food allergies and other environmental sensitivities. I fully expect that *your personal observations and common sense will convince you* of the reality of frequently occurring addictive food, chemical, and other environmental allergies.

Since food allergy and allergic food addiction are major factors in overweight, food testing will be discussed first.

Sublingual Provocative Testing

In my office, we test for food allergy by the simple, safe, and painless technique of placing a few drops of a food extract (prepared by a laboratory that manufactures testing and treatment materials for allergists) under the patient's tongue where the large veins rapidly absorb the solution into the circulation. This is known as "sublingual (sub=under; lingual=tongue) provocative testing." The allergically active substances present in the food extract are carried throughout the system within a minute or two and expose all of the body regions, organs, and systems. This bodywide distribution of food allergens often causes minireactions that clearly show the various symptoms this food can evoke when the various allergically sensitive sites that I describe as *biologic weak spots* in that particular person's body react to that food.

The same food provokes different symptoms in different allergic people, and a given person may react in different ways to each food that he or she is allergic to. For example, a sublingual test with wheat extract will give patient A a migraine headache, patient B an attack of asthma, and patient C an episode of generalized itching along with a flare-up of arthritis, patient D will become irritable and tired at first and then fall asleep or become depressed; and patient E may develop moderately severe facial edema with puffy eyelids and swelling of the upper lip. Returning to patient A, egg may cause severe fatigue, corn may evoke moderate rectal itching and abdominal distention, and milk may cause his or her hands and feet to swell. *Every patient is a one-of-a-kind, biologically unique individual. His or her allergies are different; they are caused by different substances, and each food usually affects different people in different ways.* A specific food will usually cause the same or similar symptoms in any particular allergic individual each time it is eaten.

The sublingual test is also used to diagnose allergies to airborne substances, which I will discuss further on.

Fasting

Another form of food testing, one that may be used outside of a clinical ecology test center, is the springwater fast. *Fasting is the simplest, most accurate, and dramatic form of food testing.* This is a method that I use infrequently, and I am not suggesting it to the readers of this book. It is mentioned only for the sake of completeness. Assuming that you have consulted with your doctor before beginning a fast, any physical and mental symptoms that are caused by any form of food sensitivity— including allergic hunger, allergic thirst, addictive food cravings, and allergic fluid retention—will be "perfectly" treated by fasting, because the cause of the problem, namely food, is completely eliminated when one is ingesting only pure, chemical-free springwater. Food-evoked symptoms usually disappear by the third or fourth day of fasting, and they will not return until an offending food is eaten.

The Period of Food Hypersensitivity

In most food-allergic individuals, a fast of at least four days' duration is associated with a very interesting and diagnostically important phenomenon. After a four-day fast, their bodies are much more sensitive to the effects of dietary and other environmental factors.

After the addictive food responsible for smoldering chronic symptoms has cleared from the body—whether as a result of fasting or of abstaining from that particular food—there will be a ten- to twenty-day (or longer) period of increased (or hyper-) reactivity to the former addicting food allergen. If it is eaten during this hyperreactive stage of what is now acute food allergy, there will be a diagnostically important acute flare-up of the long-term chronic symptoms that had been relieved because the food offender was eliminated. This makes the period following a fast (or abstention from a food or foods) the ideal time in which to perform a series of self-administered, single-food, symptom-duplicating ingestion tests to diagnose food allergies.

Test Meals

A four-day fast is the period of time required by the average food-allergic person to clear all food allergens from his or her body. The next logical step after a fast is to take advantage of the hypersensitive period that follows it to test the effects of each food by single-food test "meals." This "deliberate feeding test," as it's called, with one food at a time, "cooked from scratch" or eaten raw (without any flavoring or spices other than sea salt), gives the individual undergoing a series of such tests an opportunity to observe the effects of each food, uncomplicated by the effects of the many other foods ordinarily eaten together during any regular meal. Testing after a four-day fast also eliminates the possibility of being confused by withdrawal symptoms caused by foods eaten prior to testing.

THE ROTARY DIVERSIFIED DIET—KEY TO CONTROL OF FOOD ALLERGIES

The hypersensitive period follows four days of abstention from an addicting food whether or not a total fast is observed. This fact makes it possible, even without a fast, to construct a diet in which every meal (after the first few days on the diet) becomes a test of a person's sensitivity to the food (or food combination) eaten at that meal. All that is necessary is that no single food be eaten more often than once in four days. This is the fundamental principle on which the Rotary Diversified Diet— and the menu plans in this book—are designed.

My mentor, Theron G. Randolph, M.D., calls the Rotary Diversified Diet "the key to the control of food allergies," and I am in complete agreement with him. The principle upon which this method of diet construction is based is a tribute to the genius of its originator, Herbert J. Rinkel, M.D. The beautiful logic and practical usefulness of this simple technique is demonstrated daily in the improved quality of the lives of tens of thousands of food-allergic individuals, some of them overweight, whose physical and mental health has been greatly benefited by their special, individualized rotary diet plans that follow Dr. Rinkel's concept.

The diet was developed in 1934, bringing a new dimension to medical practice in the area of food allergy. Our diet, which follows Dr. Rinkel's rotation principle of eating a variety of foods at intervals of at least four days, is different from any other diet you have ever tried. It is almost foolproof, very easy to understand, and can easily be modified to meet the allergic individual's varying needs that result from changes in sensitivity that characterize cases of food allergy.

There is no guesswork involved in planning or following this crystal-clear cause-and-effect eating technique. It will show exactly how each individual food affects a food-allergic person. There are many opportunities for the rotary dieter to test and retest every available food to demonstrate its safety or the degree to which it evokes symptoms that may be within (mild) or beyond (moderate to severe) the tolerance of each individual. We will show you how to custom-tailor our diet to meet the requirements of your own unique combination of food sensitivities.

Benefits of the Rotary Diversified Diet

Despite its simplicity—a feature shared with many other great developments in the history of medicine—the Rotary Diversified Diet provides a number of important benefits to each person who has a serious diet-related problem.

First, of course, it is a highly reliable method of testing for sensitivities to a wide variety of foods with a degree of accuracy far beyond conventional skin testing or RAST tests.

Once offenders are known, it is a simple matter to eliminate all of the foods that cause a given person to have symptoms that are of moderate severity or greater. In this respect, the Rotary Diversified Diet appears to be no different from many other elimination diets, but there is a very important difference: This diet provides a well-established method for safely returning these food offenders to the diet on a trial basis after a suitable rest period has elapsed. During the period of food avoidance, it is very likely that from 50 to 80% of a person's food allergies may completely disappear and be replaced by a state of tolerance—even for foods that may have caused serious symptoms. This tolerance may remain permanently. It can be and has often been lost if the former offender is eaten too frequently because the dietary troublemaker gradually builds up in the system to a level that causes the old familiar symptoms to return. This happens so very slowly that the early phase of this process is usually unnoticed. Then the victim suddenly realizes that his "illness" has returned.

This will not happen if you are on a rotary diet. The new tolerance for former food offenders will not be "lost" because they cannot build up to symptom-causing levels when each food is eaten at the four- to seven-day (or longer) intervals that the Rotary Diversified Diet requires. The rotation of all foods, including former offenders, at properly spaced intervals is the simple but powerful key to the control of food intolerance.

The majority of food-allergic individuals will be able to eat many of their very worst food offenders within six weeks to three months (in some instances up to four to six months) if these illness-evoking foods are completely avoided in all forms during this natural recovery period. However, everyone with a serious food problem does not regain tolerance for every food that he or she is allergic to. This is due to another kind of allergic sensitivity, known as "fixed" (permanent) food allergy. Symptoms will always develop whenever food in this category is eaten, even if it has been completely avoided for several years. Some "fixed" food allergies can be successfully treated by safe medications, and some are controlled by injections or under-the-tongue drops of allergenic food extracts.

In addition to making it possible to safely and accurately identify illness-provoking foods by single-food ingestion tests, and enabling you to return many former dietary offenders to the menu, the Rotary Diversified Diet usually permits food-allergic individuals to continue eating *potential* troublemakers. Control of potential food offenders is accomplished by the properly spaced rotary intake of "borderline" foods, not presently causing symptoms but capable of doing so if they are eaten too often. **Eating a potential food offender too often acts as a series of overlapping exposures. These can add up to a food overdose and cause allergic symptoms—the potential offender has been ingested at a rate that exceeds the allergic person's ability to process and eliminate that food.** When an allergen accumulates to a level beyond that individual's capacity to handle it, the allergic symptoms that result are known as "cumulative food reactions." Cumulative food reactions resulting from allergen build-up are impossible if a Rotary Diversified Diet is employed.

Now you can see the great value of a properly spaced rotation of former offenders and presently tolerated "borderline" foods, both of which are capable of causing the various types of allergic reactions that are responsible for the overweight condition of millions of people. Susceptible people are protected from the diet situation that frequently causes acute food allergy and chronic addictive food allergy—consumption of the same foods meal after meal. "Most people eat the same few foods over and over again, sometimes quite literally *ad nauseam*. Wheat, milk, beef; corn, beet, or cane sugars; and eggs, in their many varieties and disguises, represent the monotonous basis of the American Diet."[3]

The rotation of foods in a diversified diet permits food-allergic individuals to carefully monitor the state of their food allergies. All that is required is that they do this by observing and recording their reactions to all foods. (We will show you how to keep a simple food diary.) By paying careful attention to their condition after each (single- or multiple-food) meal as they follow a rotary diet, they are involved in a continuous diagnostic process of great accuracy. From a diagnostic point of view, as long as an individual follows this diet, he or she is engaged in an unending search for the very first signs of newly developing food allergies that can be nipped in the bud before any major problems appear.

[3] Theron G. Randolph, M.D., and Ralph W. Moss, Ph.D., *An Alternative Approach to Allergies* (New York: Lippincott & Crowell, 1980).

The Rotary Diversified Diet Reveals Your "Biologic Weak Spots"

Although I have already referred to the great diagnostic value of the rotary diet as the most accurate feeding-challenge method of testing for food allergy, I am going to restate this very important information in another way to be certain that every reader fully understands this subject.

When an individual food is consumed as a single-food test in a properly constructed diet—eaten only once every four to seven days—each food being tested "stands alone," isolated from every other possible food offender in that specific diet sequence. Because of the hypersensitive period following four to seven days of abstention from the food, within a few minutes to a few hours after it has been ingested, the familiar physical and/or mental-emotional symptoms that appear will clearly show exactly what that food can do to the individual who is allergic to it.

The same food may evoke different symptoms in different people, depending on the location and function of each person's specific "biologic weak spots."[4] Thus, wheat or beef might cause intense thirst and a migraine headache in patient A; an attack of asthma in patient B; facial puffiness, generalized itching, and fatigue or depression in patient C; and a flare-up of both colitis and rheumatoid arthritis in patient D. At the same time, a given individual might have the same symptom from several or many substances that are not related to each other. Yellow food coloring, automobile exhaust fumes, tobacco smoke, a basement full of mildew, a plate of mashed potatoes washed down with a glass of chocolate milk— each may be the cause of painful blocked sinuses or frequent and urgent urination.

An allergic individual's "biologic weak spots" may involve structures throughout his or her entire body, including the nervous system. You can thus understand why **anyone with bodywide allergies could suffer from what, to many, would appear to be a hopelessly complicated disorder characterized by an assortment of seemingly unrelated physical and mental-emotional symptoms.** An illness of this type would undoubtedly be misdiagnosed as an "all in your head" psychosomatic disorder because, without an ecologic orientation, a conventionally trained physi-

---

[4]A term I coined in 1975 to describe the widely separated allergically sensitive (predisposed) areas of an allergic individual's body that are involved during the course of a multiple-site sensitivity reaction. During a bodywide reaction to some symptom-evoking substance(s), these allergically susceptible "biologic weak spots" are the affected locations. For example, along with pain and swelling in the right knee and the left hand in a case of allergic arthritis, there might also be a headache, abdominal distention, coughing, and itching of the feet as the multiple-symptom response of a food-allergic arthritic person's widespread reaction to a dietary offender such as corn, yeast, soy, or pork.

cian would conclude, after careful physical examination and laboratory studies showing no diagnosable physical illness, that the patient looked too good to have so many complaints.

However, the informed physician or patient who knows that a food offender entering the bloodstream from the digestive tract can expose all the body's biologic weak spots to illness-evoking substances will be alert to investigate this very likely possibility. The Rotary Diversified Diet, properly followed, can provide a wealth of medically useful information to help solve important problem cases by identifying their causes. At the same time, it makes it possible for an overweight person to comfortably and safely lose weight.

FOOD FAMILIES: THE BIOLOGIC CLASSIFICATION OF FOODS

There is a second principle important in the construction of rotary diversified diets that has been observed in designing the menu plans of this book, and which you will learn as you progress on the It's Not Your Fault You're Fat Diet.

That principle is: Foods from the same family are to a certain extent made up of similar substances—and must therefore be separated from each other by a day or more in order to avoid a buildup of any of those substances in the body.

What is a food family?

Botanists and zoologists classify all foods as members of either the plant or animal kingdoms. Members of each kingdom are arranged in various groups according to the special characteristics that distinguish one group of plants or animals from other groups of plants or animals.

Foods in the same family group are closely related, and share many features with other members of their particular family. In many instances, the close relationship between foods in a particular family is very clear. On the other hand, there are members of some food families whose appearance and taste are such that you would not even suspect that they are related to each other.

Compare the members of the food families listed on the Food Family Chart, Appendix D.

If you could perform a little magic in a garden where cabbages were growing, I would have you shrink them until they became one- to two-inch midgets, and when you served them to your unsuspecting family, they would be certain that they were eating brussels sprouts. The cabbage–brussels sprouts relationship is obvious even without the magic, but neither of these vegetables resembles a radish, rutabaga, or turnip, which also belong to the mustard family.

If you compare bamboo stems, cornstalks, and sugarcane, the resemblance between these tall members of the grass family is apparent, and careful examination of some other grasses will show them to be similar in construction to these taller members of the grass family. A neglected lawn that has gone to seed because it was not mowed will suggest to some that a wheat field is occupying the neighbor's front yard.

Members of the grass family do, indeed, include wheat and other cereal grains as well as cane sugar and bamboo. Dates and coconuts are members of the palm family and they grow on palm trees. Beet tops look and taste like spinach. Citrus fruits like lemons, limes, oranges, and grapefruit grow on similar trees and their cut sections resemble each other. Carrots and parsnips have the same shape but differ in color, and carrot stems and tops look, respectively, like celery and parsley.

Some of the related foods that do not resemble each other are tomato, potato, and eggplant of the nightshade family; cantaloupe, cucumber, and pumpkin are gourds; buckwheat and rhubarb; lily family members onion and asparagus; laurel relatives avocado and cinnamon; cashew and mango; almond and apricot of the plum family; lettuce, artichoke, and sunflower; peanut and string bean, both legumes; and cattle (beef) and sheep (lamb) of the bovine family.

Some foods belong to different food families but look as if they might belong to the same family. Among such nonrelated foods are lobster, shrimp and crab; chicken and turkey; scallops and clams.

Knowledge of food families is essential in planning Rotary Diversified Diets, because an individual who is allergic to a particular food may also be allergic to other members of the same food family. Related foods have certain substances in common, and food-allergic people may become allergic to foods related to their known offending foods if they are overexposed because the foods are eaten more often than every other day. In planning diets for my patients, and in creating the It's Not Your Fault You're Fat menu plans, careful attention is given to food-family relationships. It will be very easy for you to learn all of the information that you need to do a good job with your own diet.

As you carefully study the arrangement of the foods in the menu plans this book offers, you will see how re-exposures to any one food, and intervals between related foods, follow the basic principles of the Rotary Diversified Diet. Whatever diet you choose, it will show you exactly what your reactions to foods are and you will learn how much they have interfered with your previous efforts to lose weight, maintain the loss, and improve your general health. It is important for you to learn these principles and incorporate them into your daily life. Chapter 10, "Maintenance," will show you how to do this while eating less food and feeling no hunger.

SUBLINGUAL TESTING FOR ALLERGIES TO AIRBORNE SUBSTANCES

Besides the tests for food allergies, clinical ecologists have several methods of testing for allergies to nonfood environmental factors. One technique that I use often is the same as the one I use for foods—sublingual provocative testing.

Both surface-membrane and internal allergic reactions can be caused by natural airborne substances. These substances include house dust, dust mites, outdoor and household insects, many species of fungi (molds, mildews), animal danders, and pollens released into the atmosphere by trees, grasses, and weeds. Biologically active substances from these common natural allergens (which you may have been skin-tested with and treated for) are absorbed internally, especially when heavy "doses" of allergens are received with prolonged seasonal exposures to pollens and/or outdoor molds and insects, or with daily exposure to the indoor airborne allergenic particles of dusts, dust mites, insects, pet danders and saliva, and indoor molds.

Occasionally a sublingual test with a food extract will cause the patient being tested to taste or smell the dust or mold that they are also allergic to. And I have performed tests with molds, dusts, and pollens that have caused patients to become very hungry or thirsty, to crave a particular food, or have an urgent need to smoke a cigarette along with many other symptoms.

Sublingual tests are also performed to identify chemically susceptible individuals—people who respond to common environmental chemical agents that are part of our daily lives. Familiar physical and/or mental symptoms are frequently provoked by drops prepared from food coloring, preservatives, artificial flavors, automobile exhaust, artificial sweetener, pine and phenolic household disinfectants, tobacco smoke, vegetable-garden sprays, fruit-tree sprays, chlorine, petroleum-derived (petrochemical) alcohol, natural gas, formaldehyde, and other substances.

Often, but not always, it is possible to find a symptom-relieving (neutralizing) dose of a particular substance that will stop the effects of a reaction caused by that substance. The neutralizing dose may be used in the office during testing to block (turn off) the symptoms caused by the test dose of that substance. The symptom-neutralizing dose can be used to treat actively a number of allergic conditions, especially to reduce or eliminate the effects of an accidental or unavoidable chemical or food exposure. Neutralizing doses are also used by some ecologists as a treatment measure to prevent the appearance of reactions.

The ecologist must identify the major natural and chemical substances that each of his patients must avoid (and perhaps be treated for) in order to reduce their total burden of allergic stresses. This results in better physical and mental health and also decreases the intensity and frequency of environmentally stimulated hunger and/or thirst, fluid retention, and episodes of uncontrollable compulsive eating that may follow an exposure to chemicals and natural allergens in the environment.

Provocative Nasal Inhalation ("Sniff") Tests

I occasionally employ certain volatile substances in nasal inhalation tests to observe the effects of selected chemical fumes as well as natural airborne allergens in some patients. Inhalation tests bring airborne allergens directly to the allergically reactive sites in the eyes, nose, throat, and bronchial tubes.

Patients in certain parts of the United States who suffer from August–September hay fever have to contend with truly massive pollen exposure. The amazingly active ragweed plants in this country produce and release about 250,000 tons (500 million pounds) of pollen into the atmosphere each year from late summer through early autumn. Each ragweed plant is estimated to produce about 1 million pollen grains every day of the ragweed season.

In performing "sniff" tests with pollens (or molds, etc.), the allergen in the form of dried pollen grains is sniffed deeply into the nose and enters the upper respiratory tract. Strong and rapid inhalation lifts the pollen from the surface of the flat end of a toothpick (that was carefully dipped into a vial of pollen) and, with a single sniff, the allergically sensitive lining of the respiratory tract is exposed to thousands of grains of test material.

Provocative nasal inhalation tests are very sensitive and extremely accurate. They induce immediate local symptoms that clearly show what these airborne offenders do to an individual when his or her allergically sensitive membranes come in contact with them. Reproducing a typical episode of hay fever or an acute asthmatic attack by this technique provides an instant cause-and-effect diagnosis. It is the most accurate guide for determining the selection of treatment materials to be employed in each case, and it also indicates when treatment for a particular pollen can be terminated, because the sniff test no longer causes any symptoms.

In addition to the local "contact" reactions, there are important internal symptoms that result when the inhaled pollens (mold, spores, etc.)

are either absorbed from the moist nasal surfaces or become trapped in the mucus that lines the throat and are swallowed and absorbed from the intestinal tract into the general circulation. After they enter the circulation, they reach every structure in the body and frequently cause important reactions in many areas.

Avoiding such airborne allergens or filtering the indoor air during periods of increased atmospheric concentration are very helpful measures, but many people need to be given hyposensitization treatments ("allergy shots"), which are also referred to as "immunotherapy," to build up their allergy resistance. Again, it is necessary to reduce, in every way possible, the total allergic burden that may upset the delicate balance of many allergic individuals, especially when they are simultaneously being exposed to a number of symptom-evoking airborne allergens, air pollutants, water contaminants, and some potential or minor food offenders. Careful attention must be paid to each factor that has a negative effect on an allergic person, and it is necessary to make all appropriate efforts to minimize the combined effects of all of these environmental offenders.

If, after following any of the Rotary Diversified Diets presented in this book, you continue to have other symptoms you now recognize as definite or probable allergies, but they are not explained by your food reactions—especially if you have taken appropriate precautions to minimize chemical exposures and contact with airborne allergens (see chapter 5)—you may require the services of a clinical ecologist to achieve the best possible state of physical and mental health.

4

THE PSYCHOLOGICAL ADVANTAGES OF THE IT'S NOT YOUR FAULT YOU'RE FAT DIET

For me, Fran, one of the most exciting aspects of the It's Not Your Fault You're Fat Diet is that even when I am under stress, I don't eat compulsively. In the past, when something went wrong in my life, I went straight to the refrigerator or cookie jar, where I would hope to find fortification against the cruel world. Once fortified, I felt I could cope. My stress–cookie jar reaction took place almost without my knowing what I was doing. The craving was that uncontrollable.

I relied on food to make me feel good, even when I was dieting. I could be devoted to a diet—determined to lose weight—until I became upset about something in my life. Then, back to the cookie jar and the need for the foods I knew made me feel better. How depressing it all was.

When I ate the cookies, I always felt better for a little while. It never lasted long. As soon as the "beneficial" effects of my addicting foods—sugar, yeast, and wheat—wore off, the addictive cravings returned, and I had to eat them all over again. Guilt and self-blame were my trademarks. I believed lack of "willpower" was my downfall. I know now that my will had nothing to do with it. My food-addicted body had been conditioned by the misery of years of withdrawal symptoms to eat particular foods to alleviate depression. Then real withdrawal symptoms kept me eating them.

Our diet will help you cope with, or prevent, stress and depression by completely breaking your allergy-driven, compulsive-eating addiction-withdrawal cycle. You will no longer crave or react to any particular food in your custom-tailored, individual diet, and as a result, diet-related depression will be gone, because you will have eliminated its cause. Our anti-allergy diet "starves" cases of food-evoked depression, anxiety, and fatigue because they are avoidable allergic symptoms. You will be in control of your formerly uncontrollable eating and be able not to eat when under stress.

HOW EMOTIONAL DEPENDENCIES ON FOOD HAPPEN

At least 70% of the patients who come to the Alan Mandell Center for Bio-ecologic Diseases have symptoms that affect the nervous system. When we test them for sensitivities to foods, chemicals, dust, pollens, pets, and molds, we often induce brief episodes of their familiar physical disorders like asthma, arthritis, colitis, gas pains, or skin eruptions. We also find that many patients become restless, irritable, or headachy. Some people suddenly feel depressed, anxious, fatigued, or experience voracious thirst and hunger with cravings for specific foods and beverages. Still others get sleepy, confused, have difficulty articulating words, or experience blurred vision and increased sensitivity to light and sound. We have seen people become angry for no reason. One of our patients, to her horror, physically abused her children every time she had an allergic reaction. Once she understood the source of her anger, she learned to excuse herself when she felt it coming on. She would tell her children that "Mommy doesn't feel well," lock her door and rest until it passed.

At the Center, these types of nervous-system symptoms are provoked during our allergy testing. We know it is very likely that seven out of ten of our new patients will have allergies that affect their nervous systems. Our educated guess would be that seven out of ten readers have them, too. I know that might still seem unbelievable, but think about what you have just learned about addictive food allergy.

Remember that addictive allergy is a very common but generally unrecognized disorder. If you are eating foods that are causing you uncomfortable physical and/or mental symptoms, chances are you're unaware that you are ill because you are addicted to these foods. Food addiction is a double-edged sword because the same addictive foods that cause withdrawal symptoms that make you feel uncomfortable also make you feel better—at least for a while, as they temporarily suppress withdrawal symptoms. Once the food is absorbed and begins to work its way out of the body, withdrawal symptoms begin to make us feel uncomfortable and only a "fix" of the addictive food can make us feel better. On and on your addictive eating pattern goes, and higher and higher goes your weight.

The foods you are addicted to are difficult to give up, because they make you feel good—but the improved feeling is short-lived. As you perpetually eat a food that "makes you feel good," you become emotionally dependent upon that food. You recognize your uncomfortable feelings and know that your old friends sugar, bread, cake, pie, chocolate, lettuce, milk, or potato will take care of them for you. You become "hooked" on these favorite "dependable" foods that are the basis of your symptoms.

Marlene Shone, an attractive, energetic fashion coordinator, told us how much her husband hated her being overweight. She had gained 50 pounds and he was angry. He would do anything to motivate her to lose weight, and she would say, "Your mother was fat—leave me alone." They would have an argument, and she would eat to spite him. "I used to finish a whole cake. I never said to myself, 'Marlene, you are eating because you are angry at Arthur, so you are eating an entire cake.' Instead, we played a game. I would select a cake 'for the family.' My husband would argue with me because I had bought it, and he would hide it. Every Friday as I cleaned the house, I'd find the cake and be determined not to eat it. But I couldn't resist: I would begin by eating 'just a sliver,' and before I knew it, the whole cake would be gone. I'd hide the box as if I were a thief. I felt terribly ashamed and guilty."

Marlene's kind of guilt lowers our self-esteem and makes us angry and unhappy with ourselves for giving in to "temptation." Our patients tell us again and again about these feelings—the words are different, but the meaning is the same. Roxanne Mondalto, a young housewife and mother, said it very well: "I never have much hope on diets, so I just don't bother with them. I feel guilty about my lack of self-control. I'm afraid I'll fail again."

The rotation diet that we prepared for Roxanne made a world of difference for her, as the one that we will help you construct for yourself in this book will make for you. Now she doesn't have to follow a reducing diet—she only has to observe a few restrictions that are based upon her knowledge of the specific foods that cause her to bloat and eat compulsively. Roxanne eliminated bread, for example, because she was allergic to yeast. As a result, she lost weight without actually "dieting."

BREAKING YOUR ADDICTIVE EATING CYCLE

When you go on the It's Not Your Fault You're Fat Diet, your addictive cravings will disappear. After the first week on our delicious food-rotation diet, you should no longer experience the old familiar food cravings caused by withdrawal from the addicting foods you had been eating. You will not feel the old restless, uncomfortable, compulsive hunger that made you overeat. And you will understand that your compulsive eating was not your fault—you were the victim of a very common addictive disorder that had not been correctly diagnosed or treated.

As an added bonus (as if that isn't enough), our diet offers you an adventure in eating. The menus include some foods that have not been an important part of your diet, but foods that you would have enjoyed eating had you thought of them (like kiwi fruit, chestnuts, or dried papaya). We know from experience that you will feel better on our diet than you have felt in years. You are going to pleasantly rotate through a banquet of taste-tempting foods, eating each food not more than once every four days. The diet includes every possible kind of food, with enough wholesome naturally sweet foods to satisfy any sweet tooth. But the dates, fresh and dried fruits, sweet potatoes, maple sugar, and other sweet delicacies on the diet won't trigger your eating binges the way cakes, cookies, or candy bars loaded with refined sugar did in the past. In fact, as you rotate through each day of the diet, breaking your lifetime of allergic-addictive eating patterns, you will find you are less and less hungry. After the first week, food will become much less important to you, but what you do eat will taste unusually good. You won't believe how excited you can get over the flavor and aroma of *Steamed Brussels Sprouts with Crushed Brazil Nuts* or our other simple but elegant dishes.

You will learn, as thousands have before you, that by breaking your uncontrolled and irresistible addictive eating patterns that are biologically—not psychologically—caused, you will feel better without the need to compulsively eat the unwanted calories of addicting foods you depended upon for many years. Your individualized rotary diet will eliminate the physical and mental distress of your former addictive withdrawal symptoms. And when this occurs, you will be rid of the food-related guilt you never should have had in the first place.

IT'S YOUR BIOLOGY, NOT YOUR PSYCHOLOGY

As you eat your way through the first week of the diet, you will learn by experience how compulsive overeating came from years of powerful biological craving that was misdiagnosed as being a psychological need. You will eat some meals that cause one or more of your familiar aches or pains to briefly flare up. You may notice that one food causes you to feel hungry. One test meal could make you feel thirsty or tired or unexpectedly restless. You may even find yourself bloated after eating some foods. Don't worry, it is a necessary part of your education, and you will soon be in control and feeling better than you have in years.

Through it all (and it really is not bad), you will be aware of what is happening and why it is happening. The diet will evoke familiar symptoms that will prove that the foods you are eating are triggering allergic reactions. There will be many times when you will smile in recognition of your problem. *You will come to a clear understanding of all of those times your cravings got the better of you and understand why other diets could not and did not work for you—why even with diet pills controlling your hunger, you could not stay away from the foods that relieved your allergic withdrawal symptoms.* Best of all, you will know that it was not a deep psychological problem or an unmet emotional need that caused you to sabotage your diet. Never again will anyone ever be able to tell you that you "subconsciously wanted to gain weight."

From now on, you will know exactly how to plan your meals, and you will not suffer from food cravings or binges. You will know which foods to avoid—foods that previously made you feel restless, tense, irritable, tired, confused, depressed, or hungry. Your self-image and your physical appearance will change because you will know why it's not your fault you're fat.

THE "ADDICTIVE" SUCCESS CYCLE

The success you have on the diet will be just as addictive as your food allergy was. When you know how it feels to wake up in the morning and go through the day free of aches, pains, anxiety, depression, and headaches, you will never again want to go back to a place where you're not feeling well. You will gain complete mastery of your eating behavior without experiencing the irresistible hunger of the compulsive eater. Since you won't need to satisfy your addictive dependence on food to feel good, you will walk right by your previously addictive foods in the supermarket and feel no need to put them into your shopping cart.

A great success aid is the fact that if you do go off your diet, you will promptly "hear about it" from your body. You may try "cheating" and eat your old addictive foods once or twice, but I'll bet there won't be a third time! Controlling your food intake will give you a great sense of power in a life area you may have felt helpless about in the past.

For Robert Canter, a former finance professor and presently a computer systems developer, one of the greatest psychological benefits of the diet was learning that he could change his eating habits. Robert told us that he used to suffer continual attacks of voracious hunger that caused him to consume enormous quantities of food. He came to Marshall complaining of severe migraine headaches (which he later learned were caused by some of the foods he was compulsively eating). In high school and college, Robert was an extremely energetic, enthusiastic—and thin— basketball player. He ate like a giant—a dozen eggs for breakfast with huge quantities of milk, orange juice, and toast. Lunches and dinners were equally large. He recalls having once eaten five barbecued chickens at a sitting. Robert and several of his athletic friends were always trying to gain weight. They would have contests to see who could eat the most.

When he came to the Center because of his migraine headaches, he was 35 years old and was eating a little more normally—only three times as much as the average person. He believed he needed all of that food because he was still playing basketball fifteen to eighteen hours a week, though he had put on some extra weight after quitting smoking.

Through symptom-duplicating allergy tests, Marshall demonstrated that Robert was highly allergic to tomatoes, potatoes, and several species of molds. These common substances were the cause of his years of migraine headaches. (He was so addicted to potatoes that he still dreams about them five years later.)

Robert no longer has a need to exercise all the time to feel good. The constant exercise was helping to alleviate his allergies because more oxygen reached his cells and more wastes were removed as the exercise resulted in increased activity in his circulatory system. His diet is much more varied today than it ever was, and his appetite is normal.

Robert likes the fact that it is necessary to plan his meals in advance on the diet with freedom to select whatever foods he would like at any meal. He feels that planning his meals—and realizing that breakfast didn't always have to be eggs, nor dinner meat and potatoes—helped give him control of his food intake. He has found the diet an effective, self-rewarding way to change his eating habits and lose excess weight. You will, too.

THE REWARDS OF THE IT'S NOT YOUR FAULT YOU'RE FAT DIET—WEIGHT LOSS AND BETTER HEALTH

Losing weight always puts us in a good frame of mind. We feel happy about our accomplishment and the improved way we look. It becomes fun to dress up and go out—and it's wonderful when other people notice the weight loss and encourage us.

When you lose weight on other diets, you feel better about yourself, but you do not always become healthier. Our diet will improve your health and greatly increase the quality of your life. By breaking your food addiction and, thereby, relieving most of your chronic aches and pains, miraculous changes can take place in your life. We have patients who were not able to drive before they came to see Marshall because of arthritic knee pains. Today they are driving. We have patients who thought they would never again be able to play active sports, who are playing; and many of the long-term cases of depression have cleared, leaving those people free to enjoy life again.

Furthermore, you will enjoy being on the diet. It is a gourmet experience of old and new taste sensations with recipes inspired by the artistry of nouvelle cuisine. The entire diet is there for you. You do not have to deviate from it or count calories or carbohydrates; all that is required of you is some advance shopping. It is an easy-to-stay-on diet, especially with your newfound, almost effortless self-discipline.

Best of all, you will reap many benefits when the new healthier, alert, energetic, and slim you emerges.

5

WILL ALL ALLERGIC-COMPULSIVE EATERS PLEASE IDENTIFY THEMSELVES

We are going to show you what food addiction is and how it affects you. When new patients come to the Center, they are given a nine-page questionnaire to fill out. Marshall examines their answers very carefully, because in those answers he usually finds many diagnostic clues that point to the solution of each patient's specific food and environmental problems.

In this chapter, we are going to show you how to conduct your own program of self-diagnosis, which will enable you to detect and understand the nature of your food-related problems. By the time you finish these next pages, you will probably know why you developed many of the symptoms that have bothered you, either mildly or severely, for years. Once you go on the diet, you will learn if you are allergically addicted to foods, and you will have a good idea which foods and environmental substances are the likeliest causes of your weight problem and some of your other physical, mental, or emotional symptoms.

EATING HABITS INVENTORY

The first part of the questionnaire is the "Eating Habits Inventory." This consists of an alphabetical food list that includes most, if not all, of the foods that you have been eating. Next to the list of foods are several columns that need your careful attention. You are to complete the inventory by checking the appropriate column as it applies to you with respect to each specific food. Think carefully about the foods you eat and all their ingredients. How often do you eat the food—daily, twice a week, or once a week or less? Do you love the food? Do you crave it? Have you binged on it? Do you hate it? Does it make you ill? (If it does, you are probably allergic to it.)

The purpose of the food inventory is to give you an overview of your total exposure to various foods due to your eating habits, and to provide an insight as to which foods are your likeliest offenders. Only by going on the diet will you be able to determine which of your favorite foods you are actually allergic to; but filling out the "Eating Habits Inventory" before starting our diet will alert you to many possible offenders in advance.

EATING HABITS INVENTORY	Eat Once a Day or More Often	Eat Twice or More a Week	Eat Weekly or Less Often	Love	Crave	Binge	Hate	Allergic to (Get sick from)
Alfalfa								
Almond	X				X			
American cheese		X		X				
Apple / sauce / juice / cider / vinegar		X						
Apricot (fresh / dried)								
Asparagus								
Avocado								
Baker's yeast (breads and pastries)								
Banana								
Barley								
Beef (veal)								
Beet								
Blueberry								
Blue cheese (Roquefort)								
Bluefish								
Bran (wheat)								
Brazil nuts								
Brewer's yeast (nutritional supplement)								

	Eat Once a Day or More Often	Eat Twice or More a Week	Eat Weekly or Less Often	Love	Crave	Binge	Hate	Allergic to (Get sick from)
Broccoli								
Brussels sprouts								
Buckwheat (kasha)								
Cabbage								
Cane sugar								
Cantaloupe								
Caraway seed								
Carob								
Carrot								
Cashew								
Cauliflower								
Celery								
Cheddar cheese								
Cherry								
Chicken								
Chives								
Chocolate								
Cinnamon								
Clam								
Cocoa								
Cod (scrod)								
Coffee								
Cola beverages								
Corn / vegetable / cereal / popped / sweetener / starch / oil								
Crab								

EATING HABITS INVENTORY (*continued*)

	Eat Once a Day or More Often	Eat Twice or More a Week	Eat Weekly or Less Often	Love	Crave	Binge	Hate	Allergic to (Get sick from)
Cranberry								
Cucumber								
Date								
Egg (chicken)								
Eggplant								
Flounder								
Garlic								
Ginger								
Grape/raisin/juice/wine vinegar								
Grapefruit								
Haddock								
Halibut								
Honey								
Honeydew								
Kidney bean								
Lamb								
Lemon								
Lentil								
Lettuce								
Lima bean								
Lime								
Liver: Calf/Beef 　　　　Lamb 　　　　Pork 　　　　Chicken								
Lobster								
Mackerel								

EATING HABITS INVENTORY (*continued*)

	Eat Once a Day or More Often	Eat Twice or More a Week	Eat Weekly or Less Often	Love	Crave	Binge	Hate	Allergic to (Get sick from)
Maple syrup / sugar								
Milk / cottage cheese / ricotta / yogurt / ice cream / mozzarella								
Millet								
Mushroom								
Muenster cheese								
Mustard								
Navy bean								
Nectarine								
Oats								
Olive, olive oil								
Onion								
Orange / juice								
Pea								
Peach								
Peanut / butter								
Pear								
Pecan								
Pepper (black or white)								
Pepper (green, sweet red)								
Perch								
Pineapple / juice								
Pistachio nuts								
Plum / prune								
Pork / ham / bacon								
Potato								

EATING HABITS INVENTORY (continued)	Eat Once a Day or More Often	Eat Twice or More a Week	Eat Weekly or Less Often	Love	Crave	Binge	Hate	Allergic to (Get sick from)
Pumpkin and seeds								
Red snapper								
Rice								
Rye								
Safflower oil								
Salmon								
Sardines								
Scallops (bay, ocean)								
Sesame seeds, oil, tahini								
Shrimp								
Sole								
Soy/beans/nuts/oil/ sprouts/tofu								
Spinach								
Squash (yellow, acorn, hubbard)								
Strawberry								
String bean (green, yellow-wax)								
Sunflower seed/oil								
Sweet potato								
Swiss cheese								
Swordfish								
Tea: Regular Herbal								
Tomato/juice/sauce								
Trout								

EATING HABITS INVENTORY (continued)	Eat Once a Day or More Often	Eat Twice or More a Week	Eat Weekly or Less Often	Love	Crave	Binge	Hate	Allergic to (Get sick from)
Tuna								
Turkey								
Turnip								
Vinegar: Apple cider Grape wine Rye grain								
Walnut								
Watermelon								
Wheat (bread, cake, cookies, crackers, cereal, pasta, germ, oil)								
Wild rice								
Yam								
Zucchini (squash)								
Food Mixtures Bread / cake / pastry (wheat, vegetable shortening, yeast, sugar, eggs, milk)								
Candy (chocolate, corn syrup, soya, lecithin, nuts, wheat, rice, etc.)								
Coffee or tea (milk, sugar, sweetener, lemon)								
Ketchup (tomatoes, vinegar, corn syrup, sugar, etc.)								
Mayonnaise (eggs, corn or other oil, vinegar, etc.)								
Mustard								

**EATING HABITS
INVENTORY (*continued*)**

	Eat Once a Day or More Often	Eat Twice or More a Week	Eat Weekly or Less Often	Love	Crave	Binge	Hate	Allergic to (Get sick from)
Packaged dry cereal (wheat, corn, rice, sugar, salt, etc.)								
Potato chips, corn chips, cheese puffs, or other processed snacks (see labels for ingredients)								
Salad dressings (mayonnaise, vinegar, oil, seasonings, etc.)								
Sauces (tomato, cream, wheat, cornstarch, eggs, pepper, lemon, etc.)								
Soda (cola, lime, lemon, orange, sugar or corn syrup, saccharine, etc.)								
Soups and stews (beef, pork, chicken, potato, onion, celery, tomato, carrot, pepper, garlic, etc.)								
Alcoholic Beverages Beer								
Bourbon								
Brandy								
Cocktails								
Gin								
Rum								
Scotch								
Vodka								
Wine								

INTERPRETATION OF EATING HABITS INVENTORY

The inventory you have just completed gives you an opportunity to review your eating habits and your responses to all the foods you have been eating recently.

The most important dietary factors in cases of food allergy are those foods that people eat most often and in the greatest quantities. Therefore, the foods you have check marks next to in the columns "Eat Once a Day" or "Eat Twice or More a Week" are among your most likely offenders; your responses to these foods should be carefully watched when they appear on the diet. We do see exceptions to this general rule at times. There have been some instances of severe allergic reactions to foods that are infrequently eaten, and occasionally a food that may be eaten at almost every meal causes no reaction. Marshall says he is no longer surprised by any reaction to any substance in any patient.

If, while on the It's Not Your Fault You're Fat Diet, you believe you have had an allergic reaction to a food but you are not sure because you ate it along with other foods in the same meal, wait until the suspected food is scheduled in the diet again, and this time make a whole meal of that food alone. Eat as much as you want of it, so you are no longer hungry. See if this single-food test causes symptoms that duplicate the original reaction you are investigating. Always write down your symptoms in your "food diary" (see chapter 6), so you'll know what to expect when you eat the food. If you do react to it twice (or three times if you want to double-check just to be sure), remove the food from your diet for a month and then try it again, eating a smaller portion the first time you retest it. The odds are on your side that you will regain tolerance for it within one to six months, so if it still causes trouble, avoid the food for six to eight weeks and eat it again.

Binge Foods

The foods you binge on are extremely likely offenders because during a binge you compulsively eat until your desire (biologic need) to "load up" on that food is satisfied. Binge eating identifies a food addict. It comes back to the same problem: You must beware of the foods you eat most often.

Foods We Crave or Love

Very closely related to the addictive binge eating of certain foods is the frequent ingestion of foods that we addictively crave or love. The craved or loved foods also satisfy an irresistible biologic need to obtain some form of relief by eating them. Eating the craved food temporarily eliminates the craving. The foods that we crave or love are significant factors in our overweight. We enjoy eating them because they temporarily make us feel good—more alert, more energetic, more comfortable physically, stronger, happier, and more relaxed. As a result, we eat much too much of these addicting food allergens with their unwanted fat-forming calories. It is necessary for us to break our addiction to these foods by going "cold turkey."

Carefully observe the effects of these foods when they appear in the diet. If they cause hunger that you have difficulty controlling, or any form of physical or mental discomfort, avoid them for at least six weeks. Once the addictive craving for a food is broken by a four- to seven-day period of avoiding that food, you may not be able to tolerate this food in your diet. This is because you may still be acutely allergic to it although you are no longer addicted. If some foods are tolerated after they have been avoided for only a few days, they are the food allergens that cause symptoms when they are eaten too often and "build up" in the body, causing an "allergic overload."

Acute reactions to food allergens may recur for one to six months (after addiction is broken) before they "disappear"—and are replaced by a state of tolerance to that food. The tolerance will last as long as there is no subsequent overexposure to the former offender. **Regained tolerance for a former offender is a biologic miracle, but it is a fragile state and can be easily lost if it is abused.**

The regaining and subsequent loss of tolerance for a craved food is the same biologic process that occurs in narcotic addiction. This explains the famous "revolving door" through which heroin addicts used to enter, leave, and reenter the national drug treatment center at Lexington, Kentucky. After a period of abstinence ("cold turkey"), the narcotic addict would return home free of his or her heroin addiction and, unfortunately, once again be able to "tolerate" injections of heroin, with its euphoria, for a while before becoming readdicted. As the addicted state increased in severity, requiring progressively larger—and more expensive—"fixes," the heroin addict would return to Lexington through the "revolving door" to once again bring his recurring disease ("habit") under control (regain tolerance)—until the next time.

We know that it does not now seem possible that just about every one of you can easily break your food addiction and that someday you will be able to eat the foods that now make you sick, but I promise you that it can happen. If it could happen for Fran with ice cream, it can and will happen for you with many and perhaps almost all of your "beloved" foods that you will have to give up for a while. Stay on the diet, enjoy what you are eating, and before you know it your food cravings will be gone—and our maintenance diet will prevent them from ever recurring.

Foods We Hate

What about the foods you hate for nonpsychological reasons (source, appearance, etc.)? Well, where there is smoke, there usually is fire. Experience has shown that when you frown or curl your lip at the thought or sight of a food and mutter "Yuk," there is good reason to believe that you have a subtle but important "below the surface" reaction to the food—an internal response that is much less obvious than an easy-to-recognize symptom. Many years of clinical observation have convinced Marshall that "hating" is a real symptom, that food must have some negative effect or you would not hate it. Even though you don't eat these foods at all, you will undoubtedly find them on the diet and you may decide to try some of them. If you do try them, do it suspiciously, taking only a small portion the first time, and don't even consider cultivating a taste for them if you have a reaction.

Foods We Are Allergic To

If you think you are allergic to a food but are not sure, there are four helpful questions you can ask yourself. Does the food make you hungry? Does the food make you thirsty? Does the food make you physically uncomfortable in any way? Does the food affect your mental state, emotions, or behavior? If a food causes hunger, thirst, or other symptoms each time you eat it, you know you are dealing with a food that your particular biologically unique system cannot "handle" perfectly. Naturally you will avoid these foods on a temporary basis until you have fully tested them. Knowing that your body reacts that way is very useful information because it points you in the right direction toward better health.

You have the idea. Beware of foods that you eat often, love, crave, binge on, or hate, and certainly those that make you hungry, thirsty, or uncomfortable. They could be making you fat or waterlogged. Take them out of your diet for a few weeks. Retest them; check and double-check to be certain they no longer affect you when you eat them. Then put them back into your diet on a rotation basis that properly separates your exposures to these former offenders. Don't worry about their making you fat again—this will not happen unless you begin to eat them so often that you become "hooked" and reignite the addictive compulsion that caused your overeating in the first place.

COMPULSIVE EATERS' QUIZ

The second part of our questionnaire for you is the "Compulsive Eaters' Quiz." When you have completed it, you will know what you can expect the It's Not Your Fault You're Fat Diet to do for you. Your answers will show you how likely it is that you, too, like so many of Marshall's patients, are overweight because you are suffering from unsuspected, overlooked, and very frequently misdiagnosed food allergies and other forms of sensitivities. It is a detailed look at your eating habits and some of your reactions to food and other weight-affecting factors in your environment. You will find that you really are much more aware of these things than you think; you just have not spent much time analyzing them.

Answer each of the questions. The subject involved in each question is explained in detail at the end of the quiz. After you have completed the quiz carefully, read the discussion of every question you have answered "yes" to. Your answers will give you a profile of yourself as a compulsive eater (if you are one), and will enable you to understand your addictively generated emotional ties to foods and how your eating habits relate to the fat- and fluid-accumulating addictive food allergies that most of our readers are victims of.

Don't allow your answers to upset you in any way, because the simple solution to most of your problems is the It's Not Your Fault You're Fat Diet. So, take the quiz good-humoredly, without fear or anxiety, and each time you see yourself in it, love yourself a little more for being so human. Remember that at least 75% or more of all people share your food-allergy problem to some degree. It is one of the most common diseases of modern civilization. Unfortunately, many physicians are not yet aware of and are unable to properly treat this important underlying cause of the widespread physical and mental disorders that affect hundreds of millions of us—and make many of us overweight.

COMPULSIVE EATERS' QUIZ   YES   NO

1. Do you feel better if you don't eat breakfast at all? Or if you omit any particular meal?   ___   ___

YES   NO

2. At the movies, do you binge on candy, soft drinks, or popcorn?   ____ ____

3. Do you overindulge in mother's home cooking, especially when she makes one of your favorite dishes?   ____ ____

4. Do you keep candy, nuts, or some other food in your pocket, desk, or pocketbook and eat it all day long?   ____ ____

5. Do you keep certain foods in the house all the time because you are afraid of running out of them?   ____ ____
   If so, what foods do you "stockpile"?

   _____

6. Do you eat "junk food" frequently? Do you feel you can't get through a day without it?   ____ ____

7. Do you crave a specific beverage—coffee, milk, orange juice, tea, cola, beer—when you are thirsty?   ____ ____

8. Have you ever taken diet pills to suppress your appetite—and found that, even though your appetite was greatly diminished, you disappointed yourself and the doctor who prescribed them, because you could not stop eating anyway?   ____ ____

9. Does the smell of certain foods cooking make you ravenously hungry, while the odors of other foods don't affect you at all?   ____ ____

10. Do you tend to buy "more than you came in for" at the bakery?   ____ ____

11. Do you eat the same food or food combination for breakfast, lunch, or dinner two or more times a week? Daily, or almost every day?   ____ ____

12. Do you love sauces and condiments, covering much of your food every day with ketchup, mustard, mayonnaise, gravy, or some other favorite before eating it? Does your food seem incomplete without it?   ____ ____

13. Do you eat a certain food or drink a certain beverage each night before you go to bed?   ____ ____

14. Must you have a particular beverage such as coffee, tea, milk, or orange juice to start your day?   ____ ____

15. Are there particular foods you must eat for breakfast?   ____ ____

16. Is there some food—bread, butter, potatoes, tea, coffee, milk—without which your meal seems incomplete?   ____ ____

17. Do you feel particularly good after you eat?   ____ ____

COMPULSIVE EATERS' QUIZ (*continued*)   YES   NO

18. Is there any food or drink you take every day that you feel you rely on as a "perfect food"—a wonderful pick-me-up that you can count on to make you feel better and that you feel adds to your "nutritional well-being"? Is there a food that makes you feel more alert, more energetic, stronger, and/or psychologically better?   ____   ____

19. Are there seasons you look forward to because of the foods you associate with them? Do you wait for spring's strawberry picking, summer's plums and cherries, spending a lot of time picking—and nibbling—the products of your tomato patch or mini-cornfield?   ____   ____

20. Do you get relief by eating when you are exhausted, depressed, achy, irritable, or angry?   ____   ____

21. Do you get hungry in church or other places where you can't easily get something to eat and find yourself anxious to get home for lunch even though you just finished breakfast?   ____   ____

22. Do you feel uncomfortable, restless, painfully hungry, irritable, or have any other unpleasant symptoms just before meals?   ____   ____

23. Must you eat every meal on time? Will you get a headache or become uncomfortable in some other way (dizzy, nauseous, cranky, weak, restless, tired, etc.) if you do not?   ____   ____

24. Do you wake up hungry in the middle of the night?   ____   ____

25. Do you always keep some particular food or beverage by your bedside because you know that you are going to wake up in the night hungry, thirsty, or physically and/or mentally uncomfortable?   ____   ____

26. Do you have frequent or occasional troubled dreams or nightmares?   ____   ____

27. If you have been on another weight-loss diet before, have you found you could lose 5 to 10 pounds in a week?   ____   ____

28. Have you ever experienced your face (eyelids, cheeks, or lips) becoming puffy, your rings or shoes tight at certain times of day or after eating certain foods, beverages, or certain meals?   ____   ____

29. Have you found that at times, for unexplained reasons, when you haven't taken coffee, tea, a lot of soda or wa-

ter, or a "water pill" (diuretic drug), you pass considerably more urine than usual? ____ ____

30. Do you drink an alcoholic beverage at least once a day? ____ ____

31. Do you drink an alcoholic beverage at least twice a day? ____ ____

32. Do you feel unhappy or uncomfortable if you miss your noontime, late-afternoon, or evening drink? ____ ____

33. Do you drink the same drink each time you have an alcoholic beverage? ____ ____

34. Does a drink ever, and perhaps always, take away any physical or mental discomfort (such as headache, sleepiness, nervousness, fatigue, depression, itching, hives, stuffy nose, red eyes, cramps, joint or muscle pains)? ____ ____

35. Do you often or usually get acute symptoms in any part of your body shortly after drinking an alcoholic beverage? ____ ____

36. Will a small amount of an alcoholic beverage—a couple of ounces of beer or a few sips of a cocktail—give you a hangover or a lot of discomfort many hours later or the morning after, even though you positively have not overindulged? ____ ____

37. Do you get hungry while driving in traffic? ____ ____

38. In the supermarket, do you often or usually get hungry, thirsty, or sick just as you pass by the odorous detergents, mothballs, or other easily detected household chemicals? ____ ____

39. Does the odor of pine or Christmas trees make you hungry, thirsty, or sick? ____ ____

40. Do you become hungry, thirsty, or ill in the beauty parlor or barbershop? ____ ____

41. Do you feel hungrier or thirstier on housecleaning days—with their many chemical exposures—than on other days? ____ ____

42. Do you find yourself craving a snack or a soda from the vending machines at gas stations? ____ ____

43. Can you just float in a chlorinated swimming pool— doing very little physical exercise—and find that you are unexpectedly hungry, thirsty, tired, restless, or ill after your exertion-free dip? ____ ____

44. Do you crave food or drink when you are in a bowling alley? ____ ____

COMPULSIVE EATERS' QUIZ (continued)

YES NO

45. Do you become hungry, thirsty, or ill in small, smoke-filled rooms—or at work or in an automobile when people light up a cigarette? ⎯⎯ ⎯⎯

46. Does the smell of a freshly cut lawn make you hungry or thirsty, or otherwise affect you? ⎯⎯ ⎯⎯

47. Have you ever had any of the commonly recognized allergic symptoms of hay fever, hives, eczema, or asthma, or sinus or nasal symptoms? ⎯⎯ ⎯⎯

48. Are you in any way sensitive to molds, house dust, animal dander, seasonal pollens, insect bites or stings? ⎯⎯ ⎯⎯

49. Do you have any bewildering symptoms that come and go without apparent cause? These may include a wide array of problems in any part of your body: sensations in the skin ranging from itching to burning; skin blemishes; eye, ear, nose, throat, or chest problems such as itching, sneezing, discharge, congestion, popping in the ears, or frequent throat clearing; genitourinary-tract problems such as itching, urgency, "nervous bladder," unexplained pains, or frequent infections; stomach or intestinal complaints—anything from stomach rumbling to gas, irregularity, abdominal pain or colitis; muscular or joint aches, arthritis, soreness or weakness; or nervous-system symptoms like headache, sleepiness, fatigue, crying spells, restlessness, dizziness, visual blurring, mood swings, unprovoked anger, irritability, confusion, depression, impaired concentration, reading problems, spelling "errors," poor penmanship, or anxiety. ⎯⎯ ⎯⎯

50. Have you ever had the feeling or actually been told that the doctor felt you were a hypochondriac, that it was "all in your head"—or that he or she certainly would think so if you were to describe *all* of the symptoms that you have in different parts of your body? ⎯⎯ ⎯⎯

INTERPRETING THE COMPULSIVE EATERS' QUIZ

Question 1. If you find that you feel better when you skip breakfast or any other meal, the reason may be that you are acutely allergic to a food you habitually eat at that meal. If you eat a food at breakfast that you have an acute allergy to, you will regularly have symptoms within a few hours after eating breakfast. By not eating an allergen-containing breakfast, you would feel better.

Questions 2 and 3 are designed to help you further define your binge foods. As you know, if you binge on a food, it probably means that you are allergically addicted to that food. Many people think that the reason they overeat when they get some of mom's home cooking is emotional. We don't think that the reason is emotional at all. You probably crave some of mom's dishes because you were overloaded with some food allergens as you were growing up (eating her regular, and your favorite, dishes day after day) and became allergically addicted to them. But please don't blame mom; she didn't know. It's not *her* fault you're fat, either.

Questions 4, 5, 6, and 7 concern food cravings. We have discussed the foods you crave as being highly suspect as addicting foods. The likelihood is that your food cravings are your body's early warning signals announcing the presence of a developing withdrawal reaction to an addicting food. As the intensity of the withdrawal symptoms builds up in your body, you become more uncomfortable due to this allergic reaction, and when you eat the food again, your discomfort disappears, almost like magic. You have become a food "junkie."

Question 8. If it has ever happened that you were desperately uncomfortable and *had* to eat despite the fact that *you were not hungry* because you were taking appetite-suppressing pills, then you know how strong the demands of allergic food addiction can be. Even guilt and embarrassment about your irresistible compulsion to eat could not stop you. Your doctor does not know about the overwhelming power of food addiction, and this is why he or she became so very angry—"frustrated" is a better word—at you for having no "self-control" at all and deliberately going against the doctor's advice when you ate—especially at a time when you had no appetite.

But, crave no more, friends. The It's Not Your Fault You're Fat Diet will probably rid you of all of your overwhelming cravings with little chance that they will return unless you call them back.

Questions 9 and 10 are about another aspect of craving. Some cravings are evoked by the aroma of foods that you are allergic to. It is one thing for the odor of food to stimulate your appetite, but it is an entirely different matter when the aroma of a "favorite" food makes you ravenously hungry. This irresistible kind of hunger is a symptom of food addiction that is flared up by microscopic particles of the addicting food that "pollute" the air of the home, restaurant, or bakery during food preparation.

Questions 11 and 12 help you to examine your eating habits. If you are not already allergically addicted to a food, eating that food over and over again constitutes a very heavy exposure that may, and often does, lead to a state of food addiction. We will help you stop your addiction-powered compulsive eating, and like it.

Questions 13, 14, 15, and 16 concern the addicting foods that presently appear to be essential to you, because without them a meal or a day is not complete or satisfying. These foods are undoubtedly relieving some low-intensity withdrawal symptoms that you are vaguely aware of and would soon become uncomfortable from if they were not blocked (masked) by another feeding of the addicting food or foods that caused the symptoms in the first place.

Incidentally, your addiction may not be to the most obvious food you are eating. If you drink coffee with sugar and milk, coffee may not be the addicting substance; it could be the sugar or the milk that you are addicted to. In some areas of America, it could be the beets that the sugar was made from. Perhaps the yeast in your whole-wheat bread is the culprit, and you suspected the wheat.

Questions 17, 18, and 19. Feeling especially good after eating a food is strong evidence that the withdrawal symptoms of an addictive allergy to that food have been relieved. We were not designed to get a "high" from a noncaffeine food, and it is not normal to feel "a lot better," physically or mentally, immediately after eating any food, no matter how nutritious it may be. If you are dependent on any food for a feeling of well-being, the chances are very good that you are addictively allergic to that food.

Question 20. If eating a "special" food relieves any physical, mental, or emotional symptom, it is almost a sure sign that the symptom is being caused by addictive food allergy.

Questions 21, 22, and 23. If you are late for a meal or miss it completely, you may have one of the following reactions:

1. You may feel better.
2. You may feel worse.
3. You may feel the same.

If you feel better when you miss a meal, it means that you have omitted a food that would have caused an acute reaction and made you feel sick. If you feel worse, or become ill, one or more of the foods you eat daily in that meal are foods to which you are addicted, and they would have prevented your having withdrawal symptoms. If you develop certain symptoms because you are late for a meal, and these symptoms clear up after eating, until proven otherwise you must assume that you have relieved your food-withdrawal reaction by eating the specific foods you are "hooked" on.

Many people think that the headache, weakness, confusion, depression, irritability, restlessness, or anxious feelings that occur when they miss a meal are caused by low blood sugar (hypoglycemia). Marshall is convinced that hypoglycemia is really a greatly overdiagnosed and rather uncommon condition. In most cases, the "missed meal" symptoms people have are not the manifestations of hypoglycemia at all, but allergic withdrawal symptoms. We know this will come as a shock to many, but clinical ecologists have found that hypoglycemia is rare in the real world.

It is impossible to raise blood sugar levels rapidly by eating high-protein foods. Protein requires forty-five to sixty minutes to be fully digested and assimilated and act as a source of blood sugar. If you find that your "hypoglycemia" symptoms are immediately relieved by ingesting a high-protein food such as beef, chicken, pork, eggs, tuna, or cheese, you should know that these foods just happen to be very common causes of addictive food allergy, and your body could not have converted the ingested protein into blood sugar in the few minutes that elapsed before your symptoms cleared up. What you have almost certainly done is relieve your addictive withdrawal symptoms by rapid sublingual absorption of small amounts—symptom-neutralizing doses—of the high-protein foods that you are addictively allergic to.

Some people will not feel better or worse if they miss several meals or even fast for a few days. They are the fortunate individuals who are not suffering from either acute or addictive food allergy.

Questions 24 and 25. If you answered yes to either of these two questions, then you are the victim of allergic-addictive food withdrawal. After-meal withdrawal symptoms often reach a peak about eight to ten hours (and even longer) after a food addictant has been eaten. And they positively must occur with monotonous regularity during the night or in the early morning hours day after day as long as the offender continues to be eaten. When you awaken, if you eat a specific food before you can fall back to sleep, that very special food you must have is probably the cause of your allergic insomnia or the discomfort that awakened you.

Sometimes food-withdrawal symptoms are not strong enough to wake you up in the middle of the night and you will sleep right through them. Despite many hours of rest, you do not feel refreshed upon awakening in the morning. This is because you are fatigued from hours of allergic reactions your body underwent while you were asleep. You will feel better sometime later in the day when your withdrawal symptoms are controlled after you eat the food you are addicted to. If it is eaten at lunch, you will call yourself an "afternoon person" because that is when you feel well again. "Evening people" will come to life after supper because their addicting food is eaten at this time and their real day starts between 6:00 and 8:00 P.M.

Question 26. We occasionally see cases in which nightmares have been triggered by food allergy. One of Marshall's dramatic cases was a 30-year-old woman who complained that every time she ate pork at supper she would have nightmares all night long. When he tested her for pork, he found that it did, indeed, affect her mental functioning. The sublingual test with pork extract made her feel confused and depressed. After leaving the office following this symptom-duplicating test and returning to her job as a keypunch operator, she telephoned to report that she still felt confused and nervous, and had been making mistakes all afternoon.

Questions 27, 28, and 29 concern allergic edema (water retention). It is important for you to know that if you went on a total fast—not eating any foods at all and drinking nothing but water every day for an entire week—the most fat that you could metabolize to provide the energy required during those seven days would be 3½ pounds. Therefore, if you have been dieting and consuming some calories, rather than fasting, and have lost 7 to 10 pounds in a week, the weight you lost could not have been all fat. The 7 to 10 pounds of weight loss was real—it actually did occur—but well over one-half to two-thirds or more of the weight you lost was derived from retained water that flooded your tissues due to an allergic reaction that made your capillaries "leak." (See chapter 2.)

If you answered yes to question 29, then you should know that the extra urine you passed could have been fluid from your waterlogged body. You can lose allergic water weight by excreting it in your urine, through the skin, or in the breath (the lungs can evaporate surprisingly large quantities of water).

Questions 30, 31, 32, 33, 34, 35, and 36 do not necessarily suggest the presence of alcoholism. Fran does not drink "hard liquor" and never has, yet she gets very silly on two sips of wine. The reason is that she is allergic to grapes, and drinking a grape-derived form of alcohol speeds up the rate at which the grape residues in the wine are absorbed into her body. Because of this "grape overdose," she has an acute brain reaction and gets "funny."

Marshall has different kinds of reactions to alcohol. When he drank less than half a can of beer at a medical meeting several years ago, his throat and ears became very itchy, and his voice became weaker due to a reaction in his vocal cords. Beef eaten with an ounce of wine put him to sleep in the middle of a formal dinner—that was twenty years ago, and he did not understand what had happened when he woke up and dinner was over.

Alcoholic beverages are prepared by the fermentation action of brewer's yeast on sugars that are naturally present in certain foods like grapes, cane sugar, and various fruits. They are also prepared from the fermentation of sugars that have been released from the starches in grains like corn, rye, and rice. Some alcoholic beverages are even fermented from starchy vegetables like potatoes. So, to begin with, there is food at the base of your favorite drinks.

Alcoholic beverages contain residues of the brewer's yeast and the source foods they are made from, and these substances are absorbed very rapidly into the body when one drinks an alcoholic beverage. If a small amount of a specific alcoholic beverage bothers you immediately after drinking it, or causes trouble the next morning, you are probably having an allergic reaction to the foods the beverage was produced from. If every beverage causes you trouble, you are probably allergic to the yeast rather than to all of the food sources of the beverages. A few individuals, however, do react to just about every food they eat. We call them "universal food reactors."

Another interesting aspect of this problem is what might happen to you if you drink an alcoholic beverage with a meal that contains a food or several foods that you are only slightly allergic to. The offending food might not bother you very much when eaten alone, but when taken with alcohol, the mild food allergen can be absorbed so quickly that it can precipitate a severe "overdose" reaction. The same rapid absorption occurs when one takes a medication with alcohol. All of us have heard of the severe reactions (some fatal) that have resulted from the deadly mix of drugs and alcohol. We advise all of our allergic patients not to drink at all. Alcohol is a powerful food solvent and can only cause trouble.

One of our patients, Carol Bernstein, was very sensitive to the solvent effect of alcohol in carrying substances rapidly into the body. He once got sick and passed out from a small amount of a perfumed gin. The same thing happened when he drank scotch with potato chips because of his severe allergy to potato. He was also so sensitive to chemical agents, he told us, that he had a terrible reaction from breathing the fumes from fresh alcohol-based paint that had been applied to the walls of a small, closed room.

Questions 37, 38, 39, 40, 41, and 42. A "yes" to any of these questions indicates that your hunger is at least partially triggered by sensitivity to chemicals. You must read the labels of packaged foods very carefully to make sure you are not eating preservatives, coloring agents, coal-tar derivatives, or other petrochemicals with your meals. It would also be helpful if you were to empty your home of paints, paint thinners, tobacco smoke, hairsprays, deodorizers, insect sprays, nail polishes, perfumes, household cleaners, laundering agents, and other volatile chemicals. With your kind of sensitivity, it may be difficult to lose weight if you keep breathing in chemical fumes or odors that can activate your hunger.

Clean your house with a nondetergent product called Miracle White and wash your clothes and dishes with baking soda. You should buy organic foods when possible to avoid pesticide residues, at least until you can regain some degree of tolerance for the chemicals that may turn on the hunger center in your brain.

Questions 44 and 45. If these questions elicit a "yes" from you, you are probably sensitive to some of the components of tobacco smoke, or to some of the numerous chemicals used in the preparation of tobacco products. Whichever it may be, it is important to your thinness that you stay clear of tobacco. Ask people not to smoke around you, and try to avoid smoke-filled rooms. Warn people who are smoking in your presence that you might be driven by a force beyond your control to take a bite out of them if your irresistible hunger is unleashed.

If you are chemically sensitive, any exposure to nontolerated chemical substances, including those in tobacco smoke, may affect your food allergy, making you much more sensitive—more likely to react to "borderline" foods that you would otherwise tolerate. Marshall wants you to know about one of his patients, many of whose food allergies cleared up after she stopped smoking. The total stress of her allergic load was so greatly reduced when she stopped inhaling these noxious fumes that her tolerance for many offending foods was greatly increased. Half of her known food offenders no longer bothered her as long as she abstained from "this self-destructive activity that exposed her delicately balanced body chemistry to the combustion products of insecticide- and fungicide-sprayed, nicotine- and cadmium-containing tobacco that was chemically treated with taste and flavoring agents and rolled in chemically treated cigarette paper."[1]

Questions 46, 47, and 48. You may have important, often incapacitating food allergies without being allergic to airborne pollens, dust, animal dander, or other commonly recognized allergens. However, if you do have any of the traditional allergies like hay fever, asthma, chronic nasal symptoms, eczema, or hives, it is a strong indication that you may also have food allergies. Marshall has developed the concept that pollens are a form of concentrated allergy-provoking fruit and vegetable materials, in many ways like microscopic seeds or nuts. In addition, he notes that

---

[1] Taken from Marshall's forthcoming paper concerning his research projects on the allergic and ecologic factors in cerebral palsy, multiple sclerosis, polio, and the Tourette syndrome.

molds live on vegetation and on insect and animal bodies, and therefore are partially made up of these organic plant and animal substances. Animal dander consists of tiny flakes of animal skin, which he sees as tiny pieces of "meat" that you inhale and may then absorb into your system as if the dander had been eaten. It is very easy to see why people who have one type of allergy are very likely to be prone to another—they are sensitivities to substances that are essentially similar.

Conversely, anyone with food allergies is, by the nature of his or her illness, sensitive to biologic substances from the plant and animal kingdoms, and he or she may very well be affected by pollens, molds, or danders.

If you have food allergies, your food problems may be exaggerated during the pollen seasons and/or when the mold-spore count is high. You would do well to control your food exposures by rotating your foods strictly at that time. This would reduce your total allergic burden during a period of heavy exposure to airborne allergens that are absorbed into the system and often cause bodywide symptoms.

Questions 49 and 50.   We see many patients at the Alan Mandell Center for Bio-ecologic Diseases who come to Marshall with multiple-system disorders of long duration. They have been dismissed by other doctors as hopeless hypochondriacs or chronic complainers. Many have been told by conventional, mainstream physicians, who are not trained in ecologic disorders, that their assortment of undiagnosed or improperly diagnosed conditions were "all-in-your-head" types of illness.

We want to emphasize that *just about any physical or mental symptom can be caused by food allergy.* You need not have hives, hay fever, asthma, or eczema to be an allergic person. It is possible that your only allergic symptoms may be compulsive eating and fluid retention that cause you to be overweight, but chances are that you have several or many other unexplained complaints in the form of long-term health problems that neither you, nor your physician, nor his consultants in various specialties have previously understood the nature and cause(s) of.

The mystery of your poor health will probably clear up when you go on the It's Not Your Fault You're Fat Diet. When you see all or many of your familiar symptoms disappear, you will at last know the source of your chronic health problems—allergy! You have been the long-term victim of what clinical ecologists call "The Great Masquerader."

THE ALLERGIC SYMPTOM CHECKLIST

It is possible that you are still wondering about the various conditions that are included in the broad spectrum of medical and so-called psychiatric disorders to which we have been referring. The final section of this chapter consists of part of the questionnaire that is given to patients at the Center when they arrive. We have seen every symptom on the list provoked by allergy testing and alleviated by eliminating particular foods, chemicals, or airborne allergens from the diet or environment.

Go through this list yourself, checking off any symptoms you sometimes experience as well as those you have had in the past. They may well be allergic reactions. Most pediatricians are not aware of the numerous allergies that they see in their offices every day, and we are certain that you never realized what a serious problem childhood allergies can be—and that, sooner or later, some of them may cause overweight. Contrary to myth, people do not usually outgrow childhood allergies. Rather, their symptoms shift to other systems, and acute allergies often become chronic, addictive allergies.

As you go through the It's Not Your Fault You're Fat Diet, be on the lookout for flare-ups of any of the allergic conditions you checked. If you can link any or all of them to particular foods or environmental exposures, it is very possible that you will have found a way to be free of them forever—without drugs or psychiatry.

PLEASE LIST YOUR MAJOR SYMPTOMS/PROBLEMS: _____

_____

_____

_____

PLEASE CHECK ANY OF THE FOLLOWING SYMPTOMS THAT BOTHER YOU NOW, and write the letter "P" in the space for check marks if you used to have them in the past.

SKIN: itching___ flushing___ rash___ hives___ acne___ tingling/burning sensation___

EYE: itching___ red/congested___ tearing___ discharge___ puffy lids___ visual blurring___

EAR, NOSE, THROAT, CHEST: popping or ringing in ears___ frequent ear infections___ itching in ears___ excessive ear wax___ fluid in ears___ ears feel blocked/clogged___ hearing decreased___ sounds are too loud___ nasal discharge___ postnasal drip___ sneezing___ itchy nose___ sinus pressure___ nasal obstruction___ sore throat___ hoarseness___ laryngitis___ coughing___ dryness in throat___ frequent clearing of throat___ sense of smell lost___ sense of smell very acute___ sinuses obstructed/full___ sinus pain___ frequent colds___ chest congestion___ tightness in chest___ shortness of breath___ wheezing___ hay fever___ bronchitis___ frequent pneumonia___ hyperventilation___ asthma___ emphysema___

HEART & CIRCULATION: rapid pulse___ pounding___ loud___ skipped beats___ suspicious chest pain___ cold hands___ feet___ hands become white___ blue___ red___ flushing___ chills___ pale___ hot flashes___ generalized edema___ localized edema___

GENITOURINARY: frequent urination___ painful urination___ urgent urination___ lack of bladder control___ bed-wetting___ vaginal itching___ vaginal pain___ vaginal discharge___ frequent bladder infection___ "nervous bladder"___ kidney disorder(s)___ pain in penis___ pain in testicles___

STOMACH & INTESTINAL: nausea___ heartburn___ dry mouth___ burning or stinging tongue___ burning or stinging mouth___ frequent stomach rumbling___ vomiting___ diarrhea___ constipation___ colitis___ rectal itching___ rectal burning___ frequent burping___ hiccups___ abdominal pain___ bad taste in mouth___ excessive salivation___ bloating sensation___ visible abdominal distension___ passing excessive gas___ bad breath___ repeat tasting of food___ urgent bowel movements___

MUSCULAR: fatigue___ muscle stiffness___ muscle soreness___ muscle weakness___ muscle pain___ joint stiffness___ joint pain___ joint weakness___ backache___ neck ache___ arms heavy___ legs heavy___ pain in arms/legs___ swelling in arms/legs___ redness on arms/legs___ frequent episodes of "flu"___ or "virus"___

NERVOUS SYSTEM: headache___ drowsy or sleepy___ sluggish___ depressed___ anxious___ nervous___ lack of energy___ restless___ hyperactive___ crying spells___ dizzy___ poor memory___ confusion___ lack of concentration___ poor coordination___ poor comprehension___ angry and/or aggressive behavior___ feeling apart or separate from other people___ feeling that surroundings are unreal___ mood swings___ irritable___ unprovoked anger___ seizures___ learning disabilities___

CHILDHOOD: colic___ vomiting___ frequent formula changes___ persistent rashes___ chronic diarrhea___ constipation___ tantrums___ croup___ frequent/constant colds___ "growing pains"___ headaches___ stomachaches___ clumsy___ dark circles (shiners) under eyes___ poor coordination___ bed-wetting___ irritable___ tired___ pale face___ bladder/kidney infections___ unpredictable behavior___ red ears___ reading problems___ poor spelling___ poor penmanship___ slow development___ If not fed on time: hungry___ irritable___ angry___ or restless___. walked late___ talked late___ spent a lot of time sitting in an infant chair___ or playpen___ (and not on floor)___ never crawled___ left-handed___ used both hands equally well___ crawled very little___ seizures___ hyperactive___ sluggish___ tension/fatigue___ depressed___ always tired___ tired easily___

Have you ever been treated for any of the following? (Please check)

	Yes	No	What Age?
ALLERGIES			
THYROID DISORDER			
PSYCHIATRIC ILLNESS			
PSYCHOLOGICAL PROBLEMS			
HEART DISEASE			
DIABETES			
EPILEPSY			
HYPOGLYCEMIA			
COLITIS			
ARTHRITIS			
EMPHYSEMA			
HYPERTENSION			
LEARNING DISABILITIES			
COMPULSIVE EATING			
_____			
_____			

ALLERGIES

Have you ever had hives___ eczema___ hay fever___ asthma___ allergic bronchitis___ chronic nasal symptoms___ sinusitis___ insect bite reaction___ insect sting reaction___? Any of these severe enough to require hospitalization or emergency treatment at a physician's office or a hospital?
YES___ NO___

The questions and answers in chapter 12 will provide interesting information about your answers as well as your experiences on the diet and your responses to environmental exposures.

6

HOW THE DIET WORKS

Our diet is really two diets: the It's Not Your Fault You're Fat Diet itself, described in chapters 7 and 8, and the Every Meal's a Test Meal Diet, presented in chapter 9. Once you know about them, you will easily be able to choose the one that best meets your needs.

WHAT THE TWO DIETS HAVE IN COMMON

Both of the diets are based on the Rotary Diversified Diet techniques described in chapter 3. They both have cycles of food rotation that can be repeated as many times as necessary until you lose as much weight as you wish to.

Both diets eliminate foods that are "common offenders" for the first four days, giving your body a rest from those foods that Marshall and other clinical ecologists have found people are most often unknowingly allergic to.

Both diets rotate through a wide variety of foods. No food appears on either diet more often than once every four days, and most appear less often than that because we are giving you so many different foods to enjoy.

ADVANTAGES OF THE DIETS

Because both diets are based on the principles of the Rotary Diversified Diet and eliminate "common offenders," they have many advantages other diets do not have.

Advantage 1.   Your allergic-addictive eating will disappear.

With your cravings gone, you will eat less and lose weight.

Advantage 2.   As your compulsion to eat goes, so may your compulsion to smoke.

Biologically, this is an excellent time to break your smoking habit.

Advantage 3.   Just as your need for food will lessen, you may also find that you no longer have a desire for any form of food-derived alcohol.

Because alcoholic beverages are very rapidly absorbed food products, they cause food overdosing and severe addiction in the form of alcoholism. If you have been meaning to cut down or eliminate your drinking, this is an excellent time to do it. Later on, if you wish, you may test your former favorite drink and find out what it really has been doing to your body and your mind. We will not be surprised if you decide that you never want to take another drink.

Advantage 4.   You will prevent the development of new food allergies.

Many of your food sensitivities were caused by the accumulation of certain foods in your system—foods that you ate very often. When you are on either of these diets, eating each food only once every four to seven days, you will not accumulate any allergy-initiating foods in your body.

Advantage 5.   You will lose weight easily without the aid of drugs like "diet pills" or "water pills."

Your addictive hunger and allergically retained excess water will leave your body naturally (without drugs). As your allergic-compulsive eating ends, so will your allergic edema.

Advantage 6.   Many of your chronic physical and mental symptoms will clear up.

You will finally learn their root causes and eliminate any symptom-provoking foods from your diet.

Advantage 7.   You will not have to think about calories or carbohydrates during at least the first three to six weeks of your diet.

(You may never have to do so unless your weight levels off too soon.) All you have to do is eat exactly what is listed for each day, keeping in mind that portions may be reduced to match your decreasing appetite.

Advantage 8. **Not only will you lose weight on the diet, you will be healthier.**

This diet promotes general good health in every way. The foods recommended are fresh, whole, unrefined foods free of any additives or preservatives and high in vitamin and mineral content. With minor modifications, you can stay on the It's Not Your Fault You're Fat Diet for the rest of your thin, happy, and healthy life.

Advantage 9. **The meals on either of our diets are easy to prepare and to shop for.**

On the Every Meal's a Test Meal Diet, you will be eating just one food per meal, and even on the It's Not Your Fault You're Fat Diet, you can only eat ten foods a day—foods that are planned for you well in advance—so shopping is made very easy. By shopping twice a week, you can keep your refrigerator stocked with all of the fresh, wholesome foods that you need to become slim and healthy.

Advantage 10. **The diet allows substitutions from the "Eat Anywhere" list.**

If you don't like a food or won't eat it for some reason, you can easily substitute another. We have even made suggestions for substitute foods that are less costly than some of the more expensive foods on the diet, like crab, wild rice, chestnuts, and macadamia nuts.

Now that you know all the important advantages of our diets, let us look further to discover which diet is right for you.

DIET 1. THE IT'S NOT YOUR FAULT YOU'RE FAT DIET

The first diet, and our favorite, is the It's Not Your Fault You're Fat Diet. It is a luxurious diet that allows you three gourmet meals a day—wonderful, satisfying meals.

This diet is made up of ten foods a day that have been rotated on at least a four-day basis. You will not be eating any given food more than once every four days. We have carefully planned the diet for you. It is twenty-one days long and may be repeated as many times as you wish. You are given a list of all allowable foods for each day, a plan for eating the foods, and eight recipes for each of the days. The recipes offer you variety in planning your meals. Although the ten foods may not be foods you are accustomed to eating often, most of them will be foods you have had some interest in eating and perhaps never got around to trying. They are all taste-pleasing foods that most people enjoy.

The It's Not Your Fault You're Fat Diet allows you to eat a generous amount of food. You will not be hungry while you are on it. During the first five days, you may want to eat the maximum amount of each food at every meal. If you need that amount of food to feel satisfied, that's fine—you will still lose weight. But after you have been on our diet for less than a week, a wonderful thing will happen to you: You will not be uncontrollably hungry anymore. Because most of the foods you are addictively allergic to have been taken out of your diet, your body will respond by not craving those foods anymore. If you find that you need less food, eat less. The less you eat, the more weight you will lose.

The way to eat less on the It's Not Your Fault You're Fat Diet is either to eat less of each of the day's ten foods; eat fewer than ten foods; or simply skip a meal if you are not hungry for it. Sometimes there may be foods that you just don't like. Foods you don't like are easy not to eat. Otherwise, eating less may mean skipping a fruit or leaving out an oil (especially if you are eating nuts). What we do not want you to do is delete the protein from the day. Please eat the high-protein foods (meat, poultry, fish, or eggs), the vegetables, and at least one of the fruits. The rest of the foods you can alternate if you wish, eating some nuts listed one day, some oils listed another, and dried fruit another. Vegetarians are to continue eating protein-rich legumes, grains, seeds, nuts, eggs, and milk products.

Eat until your appetite is satisfied—not beyond that. The secret of our diet is that controlling allergies also controls hunger. Whether you eat all the foods or some of the foods, you will lose weight as long as you allow your new diet-controlled appetite to be your guide.

The almost magical phenomenon of having your appetite suddenly disappear is a bit of biologic wizardry. As the foods that have been causing your addictive allergies are removed from your diet, they will take your compulsive eating with them. Food addiction will be gone and with it the irresistible cravings that were part of your food withdrawal. With your former food addiction now under control, you will immediately notice that food is much less important to you. You actually can take it or leave it! After a few weeks on the diet, many people will have difficulty remembering what their favorite foods were.

Knowing exactly what you are going to eat at each meal will help you. When your apathetic attitude toward food appears, you may have trouble deciding what food you want to eat (having no particular cravings for any of them). If you do not follow the diet carefully at this time and eat exactly what is planned for you each day, you may revert to some of your addicting foods that have been old habits, thinking, "I'm not really hungry, a piece of cake or a few cookies can't hurt me. After all, I have broken my addiction to sugar, milk, chocolate, yeast and wheat." *Do not do this. It is a no-no!* Not only would you probably not feel well, but it is very possible that you may reignite your addictive eating cycle all over again. Soon after giving in to temptation "just once," you will see in your mind's eye another delicious and tempting piece of cake or a plate of inviting cookies, and again experience that old craving along with those familiar restless, irritable, empty feelings. So stay with it, have patience, lose your weight, and sometime in the future you may well be able to eat your old favorites (if only once every four days).

In the first days of the diet—the common-offenders elimination period—as you are ridding yourself of your allergic food addictions, you will also be losing allergically retained water. You will begin to lose those unsightly fat deposits that represent the unwanted excess calories you had to eat when you were plagued by the uncontrolled and misunderstood demands of your food-withdrawal symptoms, and all of those months or years of compulsive eating will soon become a thing of the past—a memory.

DIET 2. EVERY MEAL'S A TEST MEAL: THE QUICK WEIGHT LOSS DIET

This diet is one that brings many of our patients rapidly to their normal body weight. On the Every Meal's a Test Meal Diet, you eat four foods a day: one food at each meal, and one snack. You may eat as much as you like of the food designated for the meal, but you cannot eat for more than twenty minutes.

If you wish to lose weight rapidly, or if you feel you are allergic to many foods and want to find out as soon as possible which ones they are, then this diet is for you. It is the classical Rotary Diversified Diet.

Most of our patients find that they are not hungry or uncomfortable when eating one food per meal, since they can eat as much as they want of that food. **When addictive hunger is controlled, they eat less, are satisfied with smaller portions, and lose weight.**

If you suffer from severe food allergy, this diet will be a welcome change for your health. On this diet, it is possible that you will quickly find the cause of many of your "inconveniences" of life. For example, when you eat a single-food meal of tunafish or lettuce and suddenly become very hungry, you know that an allergic hunger reaction to tuna or lettuce is stimulating your appetite and is causing you to overeat. If after a lunch of wheat you feel sleepy, it will become clear why you fall alseep at your desk every afternoon at three o'clock. Carol Gaudreault, a patient who came to us with painful arthritis and got complete relief on this diet, told us that given the alternative of having severe joint pain, she had no trouble at all staying on the diet.

HOW TO CHOOSE THE RIGHT DIET FOR YOU

Most people will want to go on the It's Not Your Fault You're Fat Diet. In addition to losing weight, you will find the diet enjoyable and even fun. Each day will be a new culinary adventure. If you feel that you may have some food allergies and want to check them, there are several things you may do.

1. Review your Eating Habits Inventory in chapter 5 to see what your suspected offenders may be. When one of the suspects appears in your menu for the day, you can eat it alone as a single-food test meal and see if you have a reaction to it. If you do, take it out of your diet for a couple of weeks and try it again when it is listed in a day's eating. If it still causes symptoms, avoid it for six weeks and retest; and if this doesn't work, try again in three months.

2. Keep a food diary—any small pocket-size book will do. Write down the foods you ate in any meal that made you uncomfortable in any way. When this meal or any of the foods in it appear again in the diet, eat only one of the foods listed for that meal, and then test each of the foods, one at a time, in a series of single-food tests with a different suspect on each rotation. The record of your reactions to these foods will be very important to you when you plan your maintenance diet.

Be especially alert to the possibility of reactions on days 7, 14, and 21. These are special test days, and each day includes several common offenders that you may be allergic to. After being on the diet for a week, you may forget what it feels like to feel bad, and Day 7 can "get" you— so beware. (However, you should also remember that on any day of either diet, you may react to one or more of the foods that you eat.)

Day 14 was my bad day. The yeast, wheat, and sugar really did it to me. I became angry, bloated, and so hungry I wanted to eat everything in sight. Even though I knew what was causing it, I felt that I should have been tied down so I wouldn't be able to get to the refrigerator, destroying anyone who might get in my way. Several usually mild-mannered patients have told Marshall that they were amazed by the profound personality changes that occurred when their addictive allergies were unmasked and they had acute reactions.

HOW EACH DIET CAN BECOME INDIVIDUALLY YOU

Based on your food sensitivity, either diet can be tailored to your biological individuality. Each diet can become the perfect diet for you. As you eat your way through our diet, you may find that one food (or several) may cause edema (water retention) and that you always gain weight the day you eat it. Another food might cause you to eat or drink compulsively; and still another may give you a headache or joint pain, an upset stomach, or some other familiar symptom. When this happens, it is best to eliminate that food from your diet and either substitute a food from the "Eat Anywhere" list (Appendix E) or try a related food from the same family (see Appendix D). You may make other additions according to the rules for substitution listed in the chapters on each diet, or just delete it from your diet altogether and eat one less food that day (unless it is a high-protein food—you *must* have 8 to 12 ounces of protein a day). By doing this type of elimination, you will turn our diet into your tailor-made diet—one that will ensure your optimal health.

VITAMINS

Marshall recommends that his patients take multiple vitamin-mineral tablets. There are several brands of vitamins that are allergen-free. Look for those that are free of artificial flavors and preservatives, sugars, starches, coloring, soy, yeast, or wheat. Besides the multiple vitamin-mineral supplement, he recommends from 4 to 10 grams of vitamin C crystals taken in water or juice, an allergen-free B-complex formula, and extra niacinamide (B_3) and pyridoxine (B_6) to give added support to people with allergies. Patients with heavy chemical exposures are given extra vitamins A and E along with the mineral selenium. Chemical-free desiccated liver from Argentine cattle is also used as a special nutritional booster.

EXERCISE

The diet will give you the energy and get-up-and-go to exercise daily. Even if you do not like to exercise, you will find yourself with the energy available to do it, and you should begin to make a habit of it. The exercise you do may be in any form that you enjoy—walking, jogging (with your doctor's permission), bicycling, swimming, or an exercise program in your home or at a local health facility like the "Y" or a nearby gym. You really will enjoy getting in touch with your body.

Bill Clema, a friend who does hypnotherapy for weight loss, says he often meets resistance when he recommends that people exercise. He suggests to these people that instead of calling it "exercise," they just give themselves some extra physical activity as a part of their everyday life. Wherever they go—be it shopping, to a business appointment, or to a movie—Bill instructs his patients to park at the furthest point in the parking lot and walk to their destination. He tells me it works and it is painless.

PLATEAUS—A BIOLOGIC STANDSTILL

There may be times on the diet when you will reach a metabolic "plateau." If this happens and your weight stabilizes before you have attained your desired weight loss, there are three things you can do to begin losing again: (1) You can exercise more to burn up more calories; (2) you can eat less to take in fewer calories; (3) you can try fasting (but only with your doctor's permission) either for one whole day or for one meal a day (which is the same as deleting a couple of foods from your diet each day). One way or another, excess fat deposits must be metabolized.

But if you are like Linda Beckwith, this will not be your problem. Linda told us, "I had been a compulsive dieter, tried everything. On the Rotary Diversified Diet, I finally lost weight and have been able to keep it off—as a result of patterning of what I eat, not counting calories or carbohydrates. In fact, I can be very cavalier about what I eat and not gain weight as long as I rotate foods. It's an incredibly free feeling—it overwhelms me that I am not hungry. I feel like I've died and gone to heaven. Eat your heart out!"

Linda was able to eat to her heart's content while losing 70 pounds, and she is keeping it off. We also helped her solve a complicated long-term assortment of bewildering health problems that had perplexed many previous consultants.

Allergy-oriented rotary diets have been successful for thousands of others and they are certain to bring you success, too. Read the rules in the next chapters very carefully, and make sure that you understand them before you begin the diet of your choice.

7

PREPARING FOR THE DIET

We now know the importance of rotating our foods to avoid having an allergic reaction that will cause us to gain weight—or feel ill. We also know that eating a single food more than once every four days may be dangerous to both our health and our waistlines.

Almost everyone who enters the Alan Mandell Center as a patient goes on a rotary diet. We at the Center have had many successful experiences with this diet.

The most difficult part of any diet (this one included) is mustering the determination to go on it and stay on it for at least one week. We know that once you go on the It's Not Your Fault You're Fat Diet, you will enjoy it. It isn't boring; the diet changes every day, and so will you change each day as you lose weight and feel healthier, but remember! **IF YOU HAVE ANY TYPE OF HEALTH PROBLEM WHATSOEVER, CONSULT YOUR DOCTOR BEFORE GOING ON ANY KIND OF DIETING PROGRAM (INCLUDING THIS ONE).**

"EMOTIONAL RELATIONSHIPS" WITH FOOD

People often overeat because they are emotionally involved with a specific addicting food, not because they are psychologically dependent on eating for their happiness. We see this emotional involvement every day with patients, but some cases are more dramatic than others. The case of one patient whom we will call Alice Martin was one of the most telling.

Alice came to see Marshall because she was suffering with severe arthritis and was in terrible pain. She vowed that she would do anything to be well again. Marshall felt concerned for her, a young crippled woman needing crutches to get around. He took a comprehensive medical history that included many questions about Alice's eating habits and the various ways foods affect her. The decision was made to begin testing her immediately so she could begin at once to obtain some relief by eliminating the foods from her diet that caused her the worst pain. Among her favorite foods were eggs.

When Esther Knablin, our chief technician, tested Alice by placing a few drops of allergenic extract of egg under her tongue, Alice had a dramatic reaction. Ten minutes after the test solution was given, she suffered severe arthritic joint and muscle pain accompanied by her familiar headache, fatigue, and urinary-bladder urgency. Marshall was excited, and Alice seemed eager to learn what substance Esther had given her that was causing her so much pain. When Marshall told Alice that eggs were the culprit, Alice became quite angry.

"But I love eggs! They're the one food that makes me feel better! I wouldn't dream of giving them up!" she exclaimed. And before Marshall could explain that she might not have to give them up forever, or that she might soon stop loving and craving them, she began to berate him: "What's wrong with you? Don't you know eggs are the most complete protein food available?"

He said, "Yes, eggs are an excellent food, but your severe allergy to them is crippling you." But refusing to listen to another word, she gathered her belongings and left the office in a huff, never to be heard from again.

And that, friends, is a self-defeating, emotional response resulting from a severe case of food addiction! Alice's exaggerated emotional response to the idea of giving up her favorite "health" food is the kind of rationalization you must be on guard against—because it can sabotage your success, especially in the first week of the diet.

If you had an attachment to a high-calorie food like the one Alice had to eggs, eating too much of that food would easily cause your overweight. The It's Not Your Fault You're Fat Diet will break these emotional addictive relationships and free you to go on to optimum health and weight loss.

Share Your Observations. You may discover that you, too, are the possessor of addictive personality traits and begin to note that there are changes taking place in you because you are on the diet. As you think about these changes (in both your body and your emotions), you may want to share them with a family member or friend. Choose someone supportive who will be truly delighted with your weight loss (not someone who would be angry because you look so great and they don't). He or she may be very helpful to turn to when you're longing for that bite of chocolate bar and need someone to remind you that your craving will pass if you don't indulge it.

If you are lucky enough to have a close, supportive friend or spouse who would like to lose weight, why not share the diet with him or her and become slimmer and healthier together? We have found that when two people or more go on the diet together, it's much easier and more effective and much more fun for both of them.

STRUCTURE OF THE IT'S NOT YOUR FAULT YOU'RE FAT DIET

The structure of the It's Not Your Fault You're Fat Diet is simple. It is a 21-day rotation diet of ten foods a day. The seventh, fourteenth, and twenty-first days are "special test days." On these days, you will test the foods we call "common offenders." Common offenders are foods that are eaten more often and cause more trouble than others. The more we are exposed to a food, the greater our chances are of reacting to it.

Every meal of the diet for the first three weeks has been planned for you. For the fourth week, you will repeat Week 1—except for the special test day. The fourth-week test day will be your personal test day, used by you to test suspected foods if these foods have not already been tested at other times. To keep track of suspected foods, we are going to keep a food diary.

YOUR FOOD DIARY

Any small daily diary—or just a simple pocket spiral notebook—will do. It should be carried with you at all times so you can immediately record any suspected offender.

As you know, a suspected offender is any food that makes you feel either uncomfortable or unusually good after eating. You might feel tired or depressed. You might get that old familiar headache. Your arthritis may act up—you may even suddenly begin to feel bloated or fat, or find yourself ravenously hungry, "dying" for more of whatever you're eating.

Whatever the nature of your reaction, don't dismiss it. Write your symptoms in your food diary directly next to the meal you've just finished eating. For example: If after eating cantaloupe for breakfast on Day 1 of the diet you find you have a headache, you must suspect that the headache was caused by the cantaloupe. If you began the diet on April 14, at 9:00 A.M., then you might write in your diary, "Apr. 14, 9:00 A.M., ½ cantaloupe. 10:00 A.M.—dull headache on top of head. . . ."

If, however, you ate cantaloupe and strawberries at breakfast that day and had a reaction, both foods should be treated as suspects and recorded. Any food or foods that you suspect of causing a reaction should be eliminated from your diet until you have a chance to test them by eating each food as a single-food test meal.

At first, this may seem like a lot of work, but it is very important to you and is easy to accomplish. Because you could put on pounds of retained water or go on a calorie-loaded, fat-building binge from a single serving of any of the foods to which you are allergic or addicted, you must find out which foods they are. Remember, the purpose of this diet is to lose weight and keep it off. Set up a simple but comprehensive diary and begin to use it on the very first day of the diet. You will find the diary essential to planning your diagnostic, single-food test meals.

SPECIAL TEST MEALS

The special test meals will be very helpful to you. You will be scientifically testing, one at a time, the foods that may be causing your compulsive eating and water retention—the foods that are responsible for your weight and other problems. Once you have tested a food, if you do not react to it, the food can remain in your diet and be enjoyed on a regular rotation basis.

These test meals will teach you many things about yourself. You may learn why you wake up ravenously hungry or thirsty in the morning and cannot wait for a glass of orange juice or a piece of toast to begin your day, or why you have a midmorning slump and need a coffee- or milk-and-doughnut break to pick you up. Maybe you will find out why you feel completely exhausted halfway through the afternoon; why you snap at your co-workers at work, and your family when you get home. You will be surprised at how much information you will learn about your reactions to food. These test meals will be very instructive whenever you have a reaction.

WHAT TO DO IF YOU HAVE AN UNCOMFORTABLE FOOD REACTION

Food reactions, as we know, can cause uncomfortable symptoms. If you feel bad and are having symptoms after testing a food, you must take it out of your diet immediately and wait at least six weeks before eating it again. You may (depending upon the importance of the food to you) test it every two to three months thereafter until you find you have regained tolerance to it. Then you may put it back into your diet—but do not eat it more than once in five days, or you are likely to become sensitive to it again.

Sometimes you may feel very uncomfortable as a result of your sensitivity to the food you have eaten. If your symptoms do not begin to clear quickly and you do not have time to lie down and rest, there are several things to do to feel better.

DISCOMFORT RELIEF FROM YOUR MEDICINE CABINET

There are simple preparations that can be of great help if you are having a reaction. Many of you will not need them but they are inexpensive, and it is a good idea to have them on hand. These aids can be purchased at your pharmacy without a prescription. You will be thankful to have them if you need them, so make them a part of your next shopping list. We have had twenty years of experience with these harmless aids, and we know they work, so don't hesitate to try them.

Alka-Seltzer "Gold." At the Center, we use the gold label aspirin-free antacid that comes in a yellow box. When you feel uncomfortable enough to seek relief from a reaction, take *two* of these tablets in *two* glasses of spring water. Place one tablet in each glass, allow them to fizz, and drink them down, one glass immediately following the other. This may be repeated two or three times a day but not more than two or three days in succession. Aspirin-free Alka-Seltzer taken in this way is the best and easiest product to use. However, if you have kidney disease or a heart condition that requires you to restrict your intake of fluids or sodium, be sure to consult your doctor before taking this remedy. Again, do not take this product continually for more than two or three days, and do not repeat its use again without a two or three-day rest period.

Arm & Hammer Baking Soda (Sodium Bicarbonate). This product is probably on your kitchen shelf. Use two level teaspoons in two glasses of water (one teaspoon in each glass) instead of Alka-Seltzer "gold." There is a good chance you will feel much better within 20 minutes, but check with your doctor about the sodium. This substance does not have the pleasant taste of Alka-Seltzer "Gold."

Vitamin C, pure ascorbic acid, taken in the form of crystals, is a big help, too. Stir half a level teaspoon (always use a measuring spoon) into a glass of spring water. Drink this 2-gram dose of vitamin C every two hours for six to ten hours. If you must restrict fluids or if you have any kidney disorder, consult your doctor before taking the C. Actually, you should see a doctor before going on any diet if you have a health problem. Never take any medication, no matter how harmless-seeming, without his or her approval.

Vitamin B$_3$ in the form of niacinamide is also very helpful in relieving allergic symptoms: take 250 milligrams an hour for four to eight hours.

If you have done all these things and you are still feeling uncomfortable and cannot wait for the symptom(s) to disappear, it is time to think about taking a laxative to clear the food out of your body as quickly as possible.

Citrate of Magnesia   is a tasty laxative we have found to be very effective. Like every other remedy mentioned here, citrate of magnesia is an economical and safe over-the-counter product available at your local pharmacy. It comes in single-dose bottles, and it will taste better if you refrigerate it. We suggest that the first time you take it, you take only two-thirds to three-quarters of a bottle to see how you react to it. If this dose doesn't help, increase the dose to a whole bottle. Do not take this laxative more than once a day for three consecutive days without consulting your doctor.

Citrate of magnesia may not be the laxative to help you. In that case, there are two other laxatives to try: Fleet's unflavored, uncolored Phospho-Soda (as directed); or two to four tablespoons of milk of magnesia (Phillips', unflavored).

To speed the laxative result, you may take a five- to ten-minute retention enema. Fill an enema bag with one pint of water and one level teaspoon of sea salt or sodium bicarbonate, administer it, and allow it to remain in the bowel for at least five minutes. If one enema does not work, you may repeat it once, but do not continue to use enemas for more than two days in a row.

While it is not very likely that, by coincidence, you might develop appendicitis while on one of our diets, do not take a laxative or an enema if you are having pain in your lower right abdomen. **Call your doctor.**

TIMES OTHER THAN TEST DAYS WHEN YOU MAY FEEL UNCOMFORTABLE ON THE DIET

During the first four days of the diet, as the withdrawal symptoms of your allergic addictions are rearing their ugly heads, you may feel tired, cranky, or irritable, and all the aches and pains you've ever complained about may show up. The foods you are allowed to eat on these days do not include any common offenders, so chances are your symptoms are a result of breaking your food addictions (withdrawal) rather than reactions to the foods you are eating. If you know you are allergic to a food, omit it from your diet until you have a chance to test it after at least four days of avoidance of that particular food.

This diet is nutritious and well balanced, and you are eating fresh, whole, simply prepared foods, so the diet will not cause you to become malnourished. Your symptoms are the result of your food allergies, which are now, at last, being identified so you can do something positive about them. *Do not go off of the diet,* and do not become discouraged. The symptoms you are experiencing show how badly you need the diet. We know that well-meaning family members and friends who do not know about food withdrawal symptoms may advise you that you should not be on a diet that does not make you feel good. Believe us when we tell you that it will be well worth it. For most, the "feel good" days are just around the corner on the fifth day—and from there on in, except for test meal reactions, it can be "feel good" forever! Where else can you get a promise like that?

When you do experience discomfort, chances are that the uncomfortable feelings will not be new to you. They will be the same aches, pains, mental changes, and emotional upsets that you may very well have been experiencing on a daily basis most of your life. They are the bodywide discomforts caused by the unsuspected and uncontrolled withdrawal reactions resulting from your allergic-addictive eating. Constant exposure to foods to which you are allergic can make you feel terrible. These foods caused you to have a lack of energy, to feel tired, tense, anxious, nervous, restless, irritable, forgetful, dizzy, and they made you unable to concentrate on your work. If you have unfamiliar and/or severe physical or mental reactions, consult your doctor.

It is time to leave those weight-gaining and illness-causing foods behind and start a new day and a new you.

ABOUT THE FOODS ON THE DIET

All of the foods in the diet are eaten in rotation. You will not be eating the same food more than once in four days, and in some cases you will have a food only once every week or two weeks. The rotation consists of ten foods a day, which have been chosen to taste good together and provide a nutritious diet. Be certain that you eat the exact foods listed—pure, without anything added to them! Each day's diet includes a suggested meal plan and many recipes, so you can vary the meal plans to your taste, at your convenience. We hope you will use the recipes. Each is a simple-to-prepare, delicious, interesting combination of foods. You are certain to enjoy them.

Lunches or dinners out may seem like a problem, but they shouldn't be. There is enough variety so that most restaurants' menus will accommodate your needs. Each day has nuts, fruits, or other "finger foods" that can be packed in a bag and taken to the office. These foods make wonderful pick-me-up snacks. So plan your day's eating sequence to take advantage of the diet's built-in versatility.

PLANNING YOUR DAILY MENU

We have designed this diet to be as deliciously simple as possible. Basically, you will be eating only the foods listed (unless you need to insert a substitute food from our "Eat Anywhere" list to replace one you dislike, react to, or don't care to eat for other reasons). It is also designed to be convenient. Plan each day's eating ahead of time so you don't get stuck somewhere without the foods you need. Our suggested menu plans are just that—suggestions. On Day 1 of the first week, for example, you might want your cantaloupe for breakfast or as a part of lunch or dinner. The order in which you eat the foods is completely up to you. We provide recipes for almost any desired arrangement of the day's ten foods.

FOOD SHOPPING

For the best nutritive value, the foods on the diet should be eaten as fresh as possible. Shop every two to three days and refrigerate the food. If possible, buy your meats and fish fresh from the butcher or fish market rather than frozen (and processed) from the supermarket. Pure frozen meat or fish may be eaten, but beware of frozen meat, fish, or poultry that has been covered with gravy, dipped in preservatives, or otherwise adulterated. You want food in the purest, freshest form possible. The best way to ensure this is to read food labels carefully.

Some foods are not yet available in supermarkets and must be purchased in health-food stores. If you have a reliable source of organic foods in your area, buy as many foods as you can there, since natural or organically grown foods will generally contain fewer pesticides, insecticides, fungicides, weed killers, preservatives, or other chemicals to which you may be sensitive.

In the absence of fresh fruits and vegetables, you may use dried or frozen produce. Canned foods are least desirable. If you must buy canned foods, try to find them canned in glass containers without spices and preservatives. It may seem like a bother, but the benefits to your health are well worth it.

The diet is an enjoyable one and, unlike so many other diets, it is not boring. There are a few simple rules to follow. They are the kind of rules that are *not* meant to be broken. It is essential that you follow them diligently! Remember, one slip can put on pounds, as it did to poor frustrated Marion, a woman I (Fran) met in a cooking class. Marion confided to me that she had to keep two wardrobes because she could grow a size overnight; she never knew in the morning what size she would be. Marion's husband worried that there was something very wrong with his wife, and he was always complaining about her clothing bills. Marion didn't feel sick when she gained the weight—only fat. She told me that the only way she could lose the extra size was to go on a fast.

I was certain that I could help Marion. We worked out a rotation diet for her much like the one you are about to begin. Within two weeks, she had her weight problem under control. She found that whenever she ate foods containing wheat plus sugar—like cookies or cakes—her stomach would become distended and she looked fat immediately, not to mention the 3 to 5 pounds of allergically retained water she gained. Marion soon learned to avoid all foods that contained both wheat and sugar. She lost weight, and this time it did not return. And, lucky me, I received the satisfaction of seeing her get well—plus the bigger half of her wardrobe.

Get ready to do it right (exactly as it is written). Get set and believe that what you are doing will make you a slimmer, healthier person. And go to it!

RULES OF THE IT'S NOT YOUR FAULT YOU'RE FAT DIET

The Daily Menu Plan

Rule 1:   Follow the diet exactly as it is printed.
We have done all of the work for you; simply eat some or all of the foods that are listed. Do not omit the high-protein food of the day.

Rule 2:   You may eat all of the foods listed for each day (there are ten of them), or you may eat as few as three (one at each meal).
The amount of food you eat is your choice, as long as you do not exceed the carefully calculated daily amounts. We have provided a sample menu plan and many delicious recipes for each day's eating. If you are in a big hurry to lose weight and wish to eat less or wish to fast, see Every Meal's a Test Meal: The Quick Weight Loss Diet (chapter 9). On the It's Not Your

Fault You're Fat Diet, you will be a gourmet dieter with very satisfying, diverse meals to choose from.

Rule 3:   Foods may be substituted.

We have included a list of "Eat Anywhere" foods. (Even these, however, may only be eaten once in four days.) "Eat Anywhere" foods are listed in Appendix E and may be used freely in place of any food you do not like, any food that may not fit in with your religious or philosophical beliefs, or any food that you find you must eliminate because your test meals show you react badly to it. "Eat Anywhere" foods have two rules of their own:

a.   They should be substituted in kind (protein for protein, fruit for fruit, etc.).

b.   The food you substitute cannot be eaten again for five days.

If you are a vegetarian and do not eat any meat or fish, double the daily amounts given for vegetables, beans, grains, seeds, and nuts.

Rule 4:   A single food may be eaten in different forms during the same meal, but in only one meal a day.

For example, when using the daily recipes, if you have a recipe for french fried potatoes in safflower oil and one for sauteed shrimp in safflower oil, you could eat them both in the same meal, but you could not eat them in separate meals, because safflower oil is permitted only once a day. Other examples are cooked and raw carrots, tomato juice and tomatoes, raisins and grape juice, prunes and plums.

Rule 5:   Sea salt is permitted. Salt lightly to taste. Avoid excess!

If you are on a sodium-restricted diet, check with your physician about Morton's Lite Salt, which is half sodium and half potassium salt. It makes a delightful accent (herbs and spices will come later).

Rule 6:   You may drink as much bottled spring water as you wish.

We prefer that the water be bottled in glass, but it may be in hard plastic when glass bottles are not available. If you must use tap water (it contains many chemicals, including chlorine, that may cause allergic reactions), boil it, uncovered, for ten minutes to evaporate the chlorine, then refrigerate it or leave it at room temperature to drink when needed. Do not put "unboiled" tap-water ice cubes in it.

Rule 7:   Establish a food diary.

(See Appendix C.) It is amazing the things you will find out about yourself. Foods you are allergic to can give you many different kinds of symptoms. If after any meal you feel sleepy, restless, headachy, nervous, dizzy, extremely hungry, bloated, "spacy," or as if you have the flu or a stomach virus, chances are you are having an allergic reaction to one or more of the foods in the meal you have just eaten. (Actually, some reactions occur during the course of a meal, but they usually occur between fifteen minutes and two hours after a meal has been completed.) If you feel any discomfort, write down the foods that were eaten during that meal in your diary. Don't forget to include your symptoms and whether they are mild, moderate, or severe. Depending upon how bad the meal made you feel, you may want to consider removing the foods from future meals until you have a chance to test each one of them alone. Instead of eating the possibly offending foods, substitute other foods for them from the "Eat Anywhere" list.

Rule 8: **Meals, including snacks, must be at least four hours apart.** With some food-allergic individuals, it takes a minimum of three to four hours for them to fully react to an allergic offender. You may not know which foods are bothering you if you don't allow this amount of time to elapse between feedings.

Rule 9: **When you develop symptoms following a meal consisting of several foods—if you become uncomfortable, ill, very hungry or thirsty, eat compulsively, or experience sudden weight gain (acute fluid retention)—it is then necessary to identify which specific food or foods triggered your reaction. Make a single-food test meal of each food in that meal.**
Make a list of the foods from the meal that preceded your symptoms, and the next time any one of them appears on a day's menu, simply eat it as your only food for one meal. Use the same method of preparation as was employed for the meal that made you ill: broiling, steaming, frying, etc. Do not eat for more than twenty minutes, and observe your reactions during and after eating.

It is possible that two foods that might not bother you when eaten separately will, for reasons as yet unknown, cause a reaction when eaten together. If you find you have no reaction to each of the foods eaten alone, next time the foods appear together, try mixing two of them. Keep in mind that the cooking method might be a factor also. If you fried the first time, try broiling or steaming another.

Rules for Special Test Days

Rule 1:   Choose the one day of the week when you have the least amount of outside commitments for Day 7 of the diet.
This should be a time when you are free to eat every four hours and to rest if you should have an uncomfortable reaction after the test meal. Therefore, plan your diet in advance so that Day 7 (your special test day) is your freest day.

Rule 2:   There must be at least four hours between meals.
It sometimes takes four hours and even longer to experience your entire reaction to a given food. If you do not allow this amount of time, it may be difficult to know which food you are reacting to. When you feel comfortable after a test meal, you have found food that you can eat in rotation and enjoy.

Rule 3:   Follow test day menu plans exactly as they are written.
Eat the exact amounts of food given at the meals they are listed in. Prepare and eat the simple recipes scheduled for those days.

Rule 4:   Follow the first three special test days exactly as they are written.
Compile your list of suspected offenders. You will use them at future test meals or on the fourth special test day. At that time you will find out if you are allergic to the foods. If you are not allergic to them, you may put them back into your diet and enjoy them; the Maintenance Diet (chapter 10) will explain how. The reason we insist that you not deviate from the foods on test days 1, 2, and 3 is that these foods are common offenders, and you are more likely to be allergic to them than any other foods.

The only time you may make substitutions for the foods on special test days 1 through 3 is if you never eat that food and have no intention of including it in your diet. For example, if you *never* drink coffee and aren't planning to start now, or if you are a strict vegetarian and don't wish to test meats, or if you already know for certain you are allergic to wheat and you positively never intend to eat it—then and only then may you skip that particular test meal.

Rule 5:   On your fourth and subsequent special test days, you may test foods from your list of suspected offenders.
By saving test meals of suspected offenders for special test days, you can control which days you are likely to be having reactions. Be sure not to eat any food to be tested for the three days before and after the test.

If there are no further foods to be tested, you may, as you desire, repeat the previous special test day meals if they did not bother you. Or you may substitute foods from the "Eat Anywhere" list (Appendix E).

Rule 6: **If you find (by testing) that you are allergic to a food, take it out of your diet immediately.**

It could be making you fat—especially if your reaction to it included an irresistible urge to eat more of that food, intense hunger, stomach distention, puffiness, or weight gain from water retention. Wait at least one week and test it again. If you react again, you know you have identified a dietary culprit. Remember, this does not mean you can never eat that food again. In most people, it usually takes three to six months to reverse a food allergy and regain tolerance for a symptom-causing food. Test yourself with small amounts of your food offenders every two to three months. When your tolerance for offending foods returns, you are ready to rotate these foods back into your diet.

That's it—now you know the rules. The time has come to turn the page and begin. Enjoy and get slim.

8

THE IT'S NOT YOUR FAULT YOU'RE FAT DIET

Foods Allowed for the Day

Crab, fresh, frozen, or canned, unlimited, or substitute cod or scrod (see fish-cooking directions in Appendix B).
Avocado, 1 small
Alfalfa sprouts, unlimited
Cantaloupe, 1 small
Strawberries, blackberries, or raspberries, fresh or frozen, unsweetened, 1 cup whole
Pineapple, ½ small, fresh, or canned in water, unsweetened, or pineapple juice (8 ounces), or 4 slices dried
Pecans, ½ cup, shelled
Sesame seeds, unlimited, or 2 tablespoons sesame oil
Rice cakes or crackers (rice and sea salt only), 4
Mint leaves, fresh or dried, unlimited
Beverage: chamomile tea

Suggested Menu Plan for the Day

BREAKFAST

Strawberry Cooler*
1 cantaloupe

*Recipe included for all items in this chapter so marked.

LUNCH

Avocado-Alfalfa-Sesame Spread* served with rice cakes

DINNER

Sautéed Crab and Pecans*

SNACK

Pineapple, fresh or dried

Week 1, Day 1 Recipes

STRAWBERRY-CANTALOUPE SALAD

½ cantaloupe, seeded, peeled, and diced
10 strawberries, hulled and halved
1 mint leaf, chopped

Toss together and serve.

STRAWBERRY COOLER

1 cup whole strawberries, hulled
1 to 2 mint leaves, chopped
3 ice cubes, crushed

Place all ingredients in a blender or juicer. Blend until smooth.

AVOCADO-ALFALFA-SESAME SPREAD

½ ripe avocado, peeled
¼ cup alfalfa sprouts
1 tablespoon sesame seeds

Mash avocado and fold in the alfalfa sprouts and sesame seeds. Serve on rice cakes.

CRABMEAT/CANTALOUPE SALAD

1 cup flaked crabmeat
¼ cantaloupe, peeled and diced
¼ cup shelled pecan halves

Toss together and serve with rice cakes.

CRABMEAT SALAD

¼ avocado, peeled
1 teaspoon sesame oil
10 shelled pecan halves, chopped
1 cup flaked crabmeat
Sea salt to taste

Place avocado and sesame oil in the blender and blend until smooth. Toss pecans and crabmeat together. Add salt. Top with dressing.

CANTALOUPE PECAN RELISH

¼ cantaloupe, peeled
¼ cup shelled pecans
1 mint leaf, chopped

Chop cantaloupe and pecans together until of relishlike consistency. Sprinkle with mint.

CRAB LOUIS WITH STRAWBERRY DRESSING

½ large avocado, pit removed
½ cup alfalfa sprouts
1 cup crabmeat
10 large strawberries, hulled
½ teaspoon sesame oil

Mix alfalfa sprouts and crabmeat together. Stuff ½ avocado with mixture. Place strawberries in a blender with sesame oil and blend until smooth. Spoon onto the crab salad.

SAUTÉED CRAB AND PECANS

1 tablespoon sesame oil
1 cup lump crabmeat
Sea salt to taste
10 pecan halves

Heat sesame oil in a skillet. Add crab and salt. Sauté for 5 minutes. Stir in pecans and toss until warm.

WEEK 1, DAY 2

Foods Allowed for the Day

Turkey, unlimited
Broccoli, fresh or frozen, unlimited
Yam, fresh or canned, unsweetened, or sweet potatoes, up to 2
Currants, ¼ cup
Prunes, 8
Pears, 2 or 4 slices, dried
Chestnuts, up to 1 cup in the shells
Filberts, up to ½ cup shelled
Maple sugar or maple syrup,[1] up to 2 tablespoons
Nutmeg, unlimited
Beverage: comfrey tea

Suggested Menu Plan for the Day

BREAKFAST

Chestnut-Currant Breakfast Snack*

LUNCH

Pear-Yam-Prune Bake*

DINNER

Turkey (additive-free)[2]*
Steamed Broccoli*

SNACK

Filberts

[1]Only pure maple sugar or syrup is allowed.
[2]You can buy frozen turkey parts so you do not have to cook a whole turkey.

Week 1, Day 2 Recipes

CHESTNUT-CURRANT BREAKFAST SNACK

½ cup shelled, roasted chestnuts
¼ cup currants
1 teaspoon maple syrup

To roast chestnuts: Cut an X in the top of each chestnut. Place on a baking sheet and bake at 350° until the shell begins to peel back. Shell and quarter chestnuts, mix in currants, and sprinkle with maple syrup. Mix well. Bake at 350° for 10 minutes. Serve hot. Chestnuts can be bought in jars, already shelled, at specialty stores and gourmet shops.

STEAMED BROCCOLI

½ head broccoli, sliced into flowerets, or 1 package frozen
Sea salt
Chopped filberts (optional)

Place broccoli in steamer that is standing in a pan of water. Steam for 10 to 15 minutes. Season with salt and top with chopped filberts that have been roasted in the oven at 300° for 10 minutes.

PEAR SAUCE

2 fresh pears
¼ teaspoon nutmeg
1 tablespoon water
½ teaspoon maple sugar

Core and quarter pears. Place pears and water in a small heavy saucepan over a very low heat. Cook until soft (about ½ hour). Remove from pan and force through a strainer. Season with nutmeg and maple sugar.

PEAR-YAM-PRUNE BAKE

1 fresh pear, sliced, and 2 slices of dried pear
1 yam, peeled and sliced
6 prunes
1 cup water
Nutmeg to taste

Layer slices of pears, yams, and prunes in a small, heavy casserole. Add water and nutmeg to taste. Cover and bake at 300° for 1 hour. Uncover and bake 10 minutes longer. Delicious!

TURKEY SALAD

1 cup cooked, shredded turkey meat
1 fresh pear, cored and diced
8 filberts, shelled, roasted, and rough-chopped
Sea salt to taste

Toss ingredients together.

BAKED POACHED PEARS

1 fresh pear, cored halfway through, but whole
1 tablespoon maple syrup

Place pear in a small baking pan ¼ filled with water. Spoon on maple syrup. Bake at 300° for 20 minutes.

ROAST TURKEY

1 twelve-pound turkey or turkey parts (reserve neck and gizzards for soup)
Kosher salt or coarse sea salt

Wash turkey. Pat dry. Sprinkle generously with salt. Cover. Refrigerate overnight. Preheat oven to 425°. Wash salt from turkey. Dry well. Roast for 15 minutes at 425°, turn oven down to 350°, and cook until done (about 15 minutes to the pound).

Make a Turkey Soup for Week 3, Day 4, from Leftovers
Remove most of the meat from the bones and freeze it. Place the carcass with the reserved neck and gizzard in a pot. Add ¼ cup parsley, ½ pound mushrooms, and ½ teaspoon thyme. Cover with water, bring to a boil, and simmer on low flame for 1½ hours. Strain, cool, and freeze.

TURKEY BREAST WITH CHESTNUT-PEAR STUFFING

10 chestnuts, roasted and shelled
1 pear, peeled, cored, and quartered
Sea salt
1 turkey breast, uncooked

Chop chestnuts and pears together. Place in a roasting pan. Salt the turkey breast and place on top of chestnut-pear mixture. Bake in a 350° oven for 1 hour (or until done).

WEEK 1, DAY 3

Foods Allowed for the Day

Flounder, unlimited
Carrots, 3 large
Onion, 1 large
Grapefruit, 1 medium, or 8 ounces grapefruit juice
Dates, 8
Wild rice, up to ½ cup uncooked, or substitute oats, up to ½ cup,
    uncooked
Peanuts, ¼ cup, and 1 tablespoon peanut oil
Water chestnuts, fresh or canned, ½ cup sliced
Honey, up to 2 tablespoons
Tarragon, fresh or dried, unlimited
Beverage: papaya leaf tea

Suggested Menu Plan for the Day

BREAKFAST

Grapefruit sections (up to 1 whole grapefruit)

LUNCH

Glazed Carrots and Water Chestnuts*

DINNER

Baked Flounder in Foil*
Wild Rice with Onions and Peanuts*

SNACK

Dates

Week 1, Day 3 Recipes

BROILED GRAPEFRUIT

½ grapefruit, pitted, sectioned, and left in skin
1 tablespoon honey

Spread honey on grapefruit. Place under hot broiler for 3 to 5 minutes.

STEAMED ONIONS AND WATER CHESTNUTS

½ sliced onion
4 canned water chestnuts, drained and rinsed
Sea salt to taste

Heat a wok or heavy nonstick fry pan. Sprinkle water in the pan. Add onion slices and toss until they give up their juice. Add water chestnuts. Stir until they are warm.

GLAZED CARROTS AND WATER CHESTNUTS

3 carrots, peeled and sliced
6 canned water chestnuts, drained and rinsed
2 tablespoons honey

Place carrots in a steamer and steam for 15 minutes. Add water chestnuts. Spoon honey over the top and steam 5 minutes more. Stir well.

BAKED FLOUNDER IN FOIL

1 large sheet of aluminum foil
1 flounder, filleted
½ large onion, chopped
1 teaspoon dried or 1 tablespoon fresh tarragon
Sea salt to taste

Lay foil in a large heavy baking pan. Place fish on foil. Top with onions and tarragon. Wrap foil well around fish and seal. Bake at 300° for 30 minutes. Salt to taste.

WATER CHESTNUT-DATE SANDWICH

4 slices water chestnuts, halved
8 dates, sliced open lengthwise

Place water chestnut slice between two date halves. Eat as a sandwich.

WILD RICE WITH ONIONS AND PEANUTS

½ cup wild rice, uncooked
1 tablespoon peanut oil
2 tablespoons chopped onion
1½ cups water
2 tablespoons salted peanuts

Heat oil in heavy skillet. Add wild rice and onions. Sauté until onions are transparent. Add water and simmer until all of the liquid is absorbed (about 45 minutes). Top with peanuts. Toss and serve.

GRAPEFRUIT AND DATE SALAD

1 grapefruit, sectioned
8 dates, sliced

Toss grapefruit sections and dates together.

WILD RICE DINNER

½ cup wild rice, uncooked
1 tablespoon peanut oil
½ large onion, chopped
1¼ cups water
2 carrots, coarsely chopped
6 canned chestnuts, drained, rinsed, and halved
¼ cup peanuts

Heat oil in a heavy skillet. Add wild rice and onions. Sauté until onions are translucent. Cover with water. Add carrots and simmer until all of the liquid is absorbed (about 45 minutes). Toss rice with water chestnuts and peanuts.

WEEK 1, DAY 4

Foods Allowed for the Day

Lamb, fresh or frozen, ½ pound
Eggplant, 1 medium or 2 small
Peaches, 2 fresh or frozen, or 4 slices dried
Banana, 1 or 2
Blueberries, fresh or frozen, unsweetened, 1 cup

Walnuts, ½ cup, shelled
Buckwheat, ½ cup, uncooked
Olive oil, ¼ cup, or 8 olives
Cottage, farmer, or pot cheese, 1 cup
Rosemary, fresh or dried, unlimited
Beverage: sassafras tea

Suggested Menu Plan for the Day

BREAKFAST

Peaches and Cottage Cheese with Blueberry Sauce*

LUNCH

Buckwheat and Bananas*

DINNER

Roast Loin of Lamb with Rosemary*
Caponata*

SNACK

Walnuts

Week 1, Day 4 Recipes

BLUEBERRY SAUCE

1 cup blueberries
2 teaspoons water

Combine blueberries and water in a small saucepan. Simmer for 15 minutes, stirring occasionally. Push through a strainer. Serve hot or cold.

BANANA SHAKE

1 banana
1 tablespoon cottage cheese
3 ice cubes

Place in a blender and blend until smooth.

BUCKWHEAT AND BANANAS

1½ cups water
½ teaspoon salt
½ cup buckwheat, uncooked
1 to 2 bananas, mashed

Bring the water and salt to a boil. Add the buckwheat, lower the heat, and simmer, covered, for about 20 minutes or until well done. Blend in mashed bananas. Serve topped with walnuts. (This makes about 2 cups; for less food, decrease recipe.)

NUTTY FRUITY LAMB BURGERS

8 ounces lean lamb, ground
1 banana, mashed
¼ cup walnuts, chopped fine
½ teaspoon sea salt

Combine lamb with banana, nuts, and salt. Shape into burgers. Broil for 5 minutes on each side.

FARMER CHEESE CAKES   Preheat oven to 300°

1 cup farmer cheese
1 peach, peeled and sliced
Cheesecloth

Combine farmer cheese and peaches. Form into 2 balls. Wrap tightly in cheesecloth. Place in a small glass baking dish. Bake at 300° for 1 hour. The oven should have a pan of water on the shelf beneath the cheese to steam as the cheese is being baked. Keep water in that pan! Cool and serve with Blueberry Sauce (p. 101).

STUFFED EGGPLANT

2 baby eggplants or 1 regular-size eggplant
8 ounces lamb, ground
1 teaspoon rosemary, crushed
½ teaspoon sea salt

Parboil eggplant about 10 minutes. Cut in half lengthwise and scoop the pulp out of the skin (keeping the skin whole). Chop the eggplant pulp. Combine lamb with rosemary and salt. Add eggplant. Mix well. Stuff eggplant skins with meat mixture. Bake at 350° for ½ hour.

CAPONATA

½ medium eggplant
6 olives
2 teaspoons olive oil
Sea salt to taste

Bake whole eggplant in shallow pan at 350° for 40 minutes. Peel eggplant and chop with olives. Blend in olive oil. Salt to taste.

ROAST LOIN OF LAMB WITH ROSEMARY   Preheat oven to 400°

1 rack of lamb (about 12 ounces with bones)
2 teaspoons olive oil
1 tablespoon rosemary, crushed
1 teaspoon kosher salt

Weigh the lamb to be sure it is about 12 ounces with bones. Rub the meat with the oil, rosemary, and salt at least 4 hours before cooking. Roast lamb for 20 minutes (rare) or 30 minutes (well done).

EGGPLANT-WALNUT RELISH

½ eggplant, peeled
2 teaspoons olive oil
½ cup walnuts, shelled
6 green olives
Sea salt to taste

Peel eggplant and soak it in salted water for 15 minutes. Drain well. Chop eggplant, olives, and walnuts together until of relishlike consistency. Add olive oil and salt to taste.

WEEK 1, DAY 5

Foods Allowed for the Day

Scallops, fresh or frozen, unlimited, or substitute sole
Mushrooms, fresh or frozen, unlimited
Pea pods, fresh or frozen, 1 cup whole
Avocado, 1 small
Strawberries, blackberries, or raspberries, fresh or frozen, unsweetened, 1
    cup whole

Pineapple, ½ small, or 8 ounces pineapple juice, or 4 slices dried
Roasted cashews, ½ cup whole
Millet, ½ cup uncooked
Safflower oil, 2 tablespoons
Ginger, unlimited
Beverage: chamomile tea

Suggested Menu Plan for the Day

BREAKFAST

½ medium pineapple

LUNCH

Mushroom-Cashew-Millet Meal*

DINNER

Scallop Stir-fry*
Sliced avocado

SNACK

Strawberries or raspberries

Week 1, Day 5 Recipes

PINEAPPLE-STRAWBERRY-CASHEW SALAD

½ fresh pineapple, chunked
1 cup strawberries, sliced
1 cup cashews
1 teaspoon fresh ginger, minced, or powdered ginger to taste

Toss all ingredients together.

FRIED PINEAPPLE

2 tablespoons safflower oil
½ fresh pineapple, peeled, cored, and sliced

Heat oil in a skillet. Fry pineapple slices until they are light brown on both sides.

BAKED MILLET AND STRAWBERRIES

½ cup millet
2 cups boiling water
½ teaspoon salt
1 cup strawberries, halved

Add millet to boiling salted water. Cover pan. Simmer (at boiling) for 20 minutes. Remove from pan to small casserole. Add strawberries, mix well, and bake at 300° for 20 minutes. Yields 1½ cups—reduce recipe if necessary.

MUSHROOM-CASHEW-MILLET MEAL

½ cup millet
2 cups boiling water
½ teaspoon sea salt
1 cup halved mushrooms
½ cup cashews, whole
½ teaspoon sea salt

Add millet to boiling salted water. Bring to boil again and cook, covered, on low heat, for 15 minutes. Wash mushrooms, dry, and add to millet. Cook 15 minutes more. Place cashews on a baking sheet. Sprinkle with salt. Bake at 350° for 5 minutes. Top millet mixture with cashews and serve. This makes 1½ cups. If you desire less, reduce recipe by half.

GINGERED STRAWBERRY SAUCE

1 cup strawberries, halved
½ teaspoon fresh ginger or ⅛ teaspoon powdered ginger
¼ cup water

Place berries in a small casserole with water. Sprinkle ginger on top. Bake at 300° for 20 minutes. Serve on fresh pineapple.

HAWAIIAN SCALLOPS EN BROCHETTE

½ pound sea scallops
1 cup pea pods
1 cup pineapple, chunked

Wrap scallops in pea pods and fasten with skewers. Add to each skewer 1 pineapple chunk. Repeat until all scallops and pineapple are used. Broil for 5 minutes, turn, and broil 3 minutes more.

SCALLOP STIR-FRY

2 tablespoons safflower oil
1 cup pea pods
½ pound scallops
Sea salt
Ginger

Place 1 tablespoon safflower oil in a wok or heavy fry pan. Heat it until very hot. Add pea pods, a pinch of salt, and a pinch of ginger. Stir-fry for 3 minutes. Remove and keep warm. Place second tablespoon oil in wok. Add scallops with pinch of salt and ginger. Stir-fry 5 minutes. Toss together and serve hot.

STUFFED MUSHROOMS

8 large fresh mushrooms
2 tablespoons safflower oil
6 cashews
1 teaspoon fresh ginger
Sea salt to taste

Wash mushrooms and remove stems. Heat oil in a skillet and sauté mushroom caps with a little salt. Remove mushroom caps and set aside. Chop mushroom stems, cashews, and ginger together until fine. Add the mixture to the oil in the pan, season with salt, and sauté for 2 minutes. Remove from skillet and stuff mushroom caps with mixture. Place mushrooms on a baking sheet and bake at 350° for 10 minutes.

WEEK 1, DAY 6

Foods Allowed for the Day

Salmon or swordfish, unlimited, or substitute turbot, fresh or frozen (see fish-cooking instructions in Appendix B).
Spinach, fresh or frozen, unlimited
Brussels sprouts, fresh or frozen, unlimited
Bacon, nitrate-free, 5 slices, and 1 tablespoon bacon fat
Apricots, 2 fresh, or 4 slices dried, and 1 tablespoon apricot oil
Grapes, 1 cup, or raisins, up to ½ cup
Lemons, unlimited
Brazil nuts, ½ cup whole
Eggs, 3

Pepper, unlimited
Beverage: spearmint tea

Suggested Menu Plan for the Day

BREAKFAST

Spinach Omelet* with bacon

LUNCH

Brussels Sprouts and Roasted Brazil Nuts*

DINNER

Poached Salmon and Grapes with Lemon Sauce*

SNACK

Apricots, 2 fresh, or 4 slices, dried

Week 1, Day 6 Recipes

DEVILED SALMON EGGS

3 hard-boiled eggs, shelled
1 can waterpacked salmon, drained; or 2 ounces fresh, poached and drained
Juice of ½ lemon
Sea salt and pepper to taste

Cut eggs in half lengthwise. Remove yolks and mash them with salmon, lemon juice, salt, and pepper. Spoon yolk mixture into cavity of egg whites.

SCRAMBLED EGGS AND APRICOTS

4 dried apricots
3 eggs
2 teaspoons apricot oil (optional)

Soak dried apricots in water until soft. Pour off water. Cook apricots on low flame for 20 minutes, stirring often. Combine apricots with eggs. Beat well. Heat apricot oil in a small skillet or use nonstick pan. Add egg-apricot mixture and scramble until cooked.

SPINACH AND BACON OMELET

3 eggs
½ pound fresh spinach or ¼ box frozen
5 slices bacon
1 tablespoon bacon fat
Sea salt and pepper to taste

Beat eggs. Cook spinach in a small amount of salted water for 5 minutes. Drain well. Rough-chop and add spinach to eggs. Sprinkle with salt and pepper. Heat a fry pan. Fry bacon and drain well. Reserve 1 tablespoon bacon fat in pan. Place egg mixture in pan. Crumble bacon over eggs. Cook over a low heat, lifting edges with spatula so uncooked omelet can flow under. Cook until top begins to look dry. Lift edge and fold omelet in half. Remove from pan.

SALMON CAVIAR WITH CHOPPED EGGS AND LEMON

1 jar salmon caviar
2 hard-boiled eggs, chopped
¼ lemon cut into wedges
Pepper to taste

Toss together all ingredients except lemon. Garnish with lemon.

POACHED SALMON AND GRAPES WITH LEMON SAUCE

½ pound salmon steak about 1 inch thick
Sea salt
1 cup white seedless grapes
Juice of 1 lemon

Wrap salmon in cheesecloth to make it easier to lift out of the water in one piece. Half-fill a skillet with salted water and bring to a boil. Place the salmon in the water, bring to a boil again, and allow salmon to poach for 12 minutes. When the salmon has cooked for 6 minutes, add the grapes. Remove salmon and grapes from water and unwrap salmon steak. Combine lemon juice and salt. Serve with the salmon.

GRAPE SODA

1 cup seedless grapes
¼ cup club soda or mineral water

Push grapes through a strainer. Add club soda or mineral water. Stir well.

BRUSSELS SPROUTS AND ROASTED BRAZIL NUTS

1 dozen fresh brussels sprouts or 1 package frozen
½ cup Brazil nuts
Lemon juice and sea salt to taste

Cook frozen brussels sprouts according to package directions, or steam fresh brussels sprouts about ½ hour until soft. Add Brazil nuts that have been roasted in a 300° oven for 10 minutes and chopped. Add salt and lemon juice.

TRAIL MIX

4 slices dried apricots
½ cup raisins
½ cup Brazil nuts

Mix together well. Makes a great lunch.

WEEK 1, DAY 7

Special Test Day

Foods Allowed for the Day

Beef, ½ pound[3]
Figs, fresh or dried, 4
Watermelon, unlimited, or honeydew melon, fresh or frozen
Potatoes, 1 to 2
Corn, up to 3 ears; or Niblets, fresh or frozen, unlimited; or corn oil, 2
    tablespoons; or popcorn (½ cup unpopped)
Parsley, fresh or dried, unlimited
Pecans, ½ cup shelled
Honey, 2 tablespoons
Any commercial tea

Today the following foods MUST be eaten at each meal:

BREAKFAST

Watermelon or honeydew (unlimited)

[3] Vegetarians may substitute a vegetable in rotation for beef.

LUNCH

3 ears of corn (or Niblets packed in water)
½ cup popcorn (unpopped) with Parsley Corn Oil*

DINNER

Roast Beef with Oven-Browned Potatoes*
Pecans
Tea with honey

SNACK

Figs

Week 1, Day 7 Recipes

PARSLEY CORN OIL

1 tablespoon fresh parsley
Sea salt to taste
2 tablespoons corn oil, heated

Roast parsley in preheated 350° oven for 5 minutes. Chop fine. Add parsley and salt to warm corn oil. Pour over popcorn. Serve.

ROAST BEEF WITH OVEN-BROWNED POTATOES   Preheat oven to 325°

1 small roast beef (about 1½ pounds, boned)
2 potatoes, peeled and washed
Sea salt to taste

Place roast in the center of a medium-size baking pan. Slice potatoes very thin and place around the roast. Salt to taste. Roast in 325° oven for 35 minutes, turning potatoes once.

WEEK 2, DAY 1

Foods Allowed for the Day

Shrimp, fresh or frozen, unlimited, or substitute haddock, fresh or frozen
    (see fish-cooking instructions in Appendix B).

Tuna, fresh or canned in water

Peas, sweet, 1 cup fresh or frozen

Tomatoes, fresh, 2, or 8-ounce can tomato sauce without sugar, or 8 ounces tomato juice, unsweetened

Carrots, 3

Papaya, 1 fresh, or 4 slices dried

Blueberries, fresh or frozen, 1 cup

Macadamia nuts, ½ cup shelled, or substitute filberts

Sesame oil, ¼ cup, or sesame seeds, ¼ cup

Dill, fresh or dried, unlimited

Beverage: ginseng tea.

Suggested Menu Plan for the Day

BREAKFAST

Papaya with Blueberry Sauce*

LUNCH

Tuna-Carrot-Tomato Casserole*

DINNER

Stir-fried Shrimp and Peas*

SNACK

Macadamia nuts

Week 2, Day 1 Recipes

TOMATO SAUCE

2 fresh tomatoes
⅛ cup water
¼ teaspoon dried dill or ½ teaspoon fresh
½ cup peas, fresh or frozen
Sea salt to taste

Place all ingredients in a small heavy saucepan. Bring to a boil, then lower heat and simmer gently for ½ hour, uncovered. Serve as a dip for shrimp.

STEWED TOMATOES WITH DILL

2 tomatoes
½ teaspoon dried dill or 1 teaspoon fresh dill leaves, chopped
Sea salt to taste

Quarter tomatoes. Sprinkle with dill. Place in a small saucepan and simmer gently for ½ hour. Salt to taste.

TUNA-CARROT-TOMATO CASSEROLE   Preheat oven to 350°

1 can water-packed tuna
2 carrots, grated
4 ounces tomato sauce
¼ teaspoon dill
Sea salt to taste

Drain tuna. Mix with carrots, tomato sauce, dill, and salt. Bake in a small oven-proof dish for 20 minutes in a 350° oven.

STIR-FRIED SHRIMP AND PEAS

8 jumbo shrimp
1 cup peas
1 to 2 tablespoons sesame seeds
2 tablespoons sesame oil
Sea salt to taste

Peel and devein raw shrimp. Pour 1 tablespoon of the oil into a wok or heavy fry pan and allow it to get hot. Add peas with a pinch of salt. Stir-fry for 3 to 5 minutes (until cooked). Remove from wok and keep warm. Add last tablespoon of oil to wok. Allow it to get hot, and put shrimp in. Stir-fry shrimp for about 7 minutes, or until done. Return peas to the wok. Add sesame seeds, toss well, and serve immediately.

STUFFED TOMATOES

2 tomatoes
6 medium shrimp, cooked and cleaned
½ cup peas, fresh or frozen
Sea salt and dill to taste

Core and scoop out tomatoes. Do not go through to the bottom of tomato. Cook frozen peas according to package directions. Steam fresh peas for 5 to 10 minutes (until done). Chop shrimp and peas together. Combine with tomato pulp, salt, and dill. Spoon mixture into tomato skins. Serve cold.

POTTED SHRIMP AND TOMATOES WITH DILL

10 shrimp
1 recipe Stewed Tomatoes with Dill (p. 112)
Sea salt to taste

Place shrimp and the Stewed Tomatoes with Dill in a heavy saucepan. Bring to a boil. Lower heat and simmer for 10 minutes.

PEA SOUP

1 cup shelled sweet peas
1 recipe Stewed Tomatoes with Dill (p. 112)
½ cup water
Sea salt to taste

Put shelled peas in small heavy saucepan. Add water and Stewed Tomatoes with Dill. Simmer over low heat for 45 minutes. Add salt to taste. Blend in blender until smooth. Reheat and serve.

PAPAYA WITH BLUEBERRY SAUCE

One recipe Blueberry Sauce (p. 101)
1 fresh papaya or 4 slices dried that have been soaked in water
½ cup whole blueberries

Dice papaya. Mix sauce with papaya. Top with whole blueberries.

WEEK 2, DAY 2

Foods Allowed for the Day

Fillet of sole, fresh or frozen, unlimited
Lettuce, unlimited
Cucumbers, 2
Radishes, unlimited
Apples, 2, or 4 slices dried
Kiwi fruit (Chinese gooseberries), 2
Almonds, ½ cup, shelled, and 1 tablespoon almond oil
Brown rice, 1 cup uncooked
Safflower oil, ¼ cup
Vinegar, ¼ cup
Beverage: comfrey tea

Suggested Menu Plan for the Day

BREAKFAST

Applesauce* or 2 apples

LUNCH

Brown Rice with Almonds and Cucumbers*

DINNER

Baked Fillet of Sole* in lettuce leaves
Lettuce-Radish Salad with Oil and Vinegar Dressing*

SNACK

Toasted Almonds*

Week 2, Day 2 Recipes

RICE AND APPLE LETTUCE ROLLS

½ cup brown rice
1 cup plus 2 tablespoons water
2 apples, peeled, cored, and diced fine
¼ cup almonds, chopped
8 large lettuce leaves
Sea salt

Place rice in small saucepan with water. Bring to a boil. Reduce heat and simmer, covered, for ½ hour. Mix in diced apples and almonds. Salt to taste. Divide mixture among the lettuce leaves. Roll them up.

CUCUMBER, ALMOND, MUSTARD RELISH

1 cucumber, washed well
1 teaspoon vinegar
4 radishes
¼ cup almonds

Slice cucumber to the thinness of half-dollars. Sprinkle with vinegar. Allow to sit for 20 minutes. Add radishes and almonds. Chop to relish consistency.

APPLESAUCE

2 apples, cored and quartered
2 tablespoons water

Cook apples very slowly in a heavy saucepan for about 20 minutes or until done. Push through a strainer (or use a Foley mill). Refrigerate.

MARINATED CUCUMBERS   Must be prepared the day before.

2 cucumbers
2 tablespoons vinegar
1 teaspoon white horseradish

Wash and slice cucumbers (peeling optional). Dry them well. Mix vinegar and horseradish and marinate cucumbers in horseradish mixture overnight.

BAKED FILLET OF SOLE IN LETTUCE LEAVES   Preheat oven to 350°

Fillet of sole
Sea salt
Enough lettuce leaves to cover sole

Lay lettuce leaves in baking pan. Top with fish. Sprinkle with sea salt. Top with more lettuce leaves. Bake at 350° for 20 minutes.

LETTUCE-RADISH SALAD WITH OIL AND VINEGAR DRESSING

Lettuce, as much as you wish of any kind you wish
10 radishes, chopped

To make dressing, place the following in a small screw-top jar:
2 tablespoons vinegar
4 tablespoons safflower oil
⅛ teaspoon sea salt

Shake well. Refrigerate.

FILLET OF SOLE AMANDINE   Preheat oven to 350°

½ pound fillet of sole
¼ cup almonds, whole or halved
Sea salt to taste
1 to 2 tablespoons safflower oil

Place fillet of sole in baking dish. Top with almonds and salt. Sprinkle with oil. Bake at 350° for 15 minutes.

BROWN RICE WITH ALMONDS AND CUCUMBERS

1 cup brown rice
2 tablespoons almond oil
2½ cups water
¼ teaspoon sea salt
¼ cup almonds
1 to 2 cucumbers, peeled and diced

In a small heavy saucepan, sauté rice in almond oil for 3 minutes. Add water and salt. Bring to boil. Cover and simmer on low heat for ½ hour or until rice is cooked. Add cucumbers and almonds. Toss and serve.

WEEK 2, DAY 3

Foods Allowed for the Day

Beef or calf's liver, fresh or frozen, unlimited, and 2 tablespoons butter, or substitute fresh or frozen trout, unlimited (see fish-cooking directions in Appendix B).
Onion, 1 large
String beans, fresh or frozen, unlimited
Peppers, sweet green or red, 2
Bananas, 1 or 2
Strawberries, blackberries, or raspberries, fresh or frozen, unsweetened, 1 cup whole
Pine nuts, ¼ cup, or substitute hickory
Coconut, ¼ fresh or ¼ cup grated or 2 tablespoons dried
Buckwheat, ½ cup uncooked
Nutmeg, unlimited
Beverage: sassafras tea

Suggested Menu Plan for the Day

BREAKFAST

2 bananas

LUNCH

Buckwheat and Peppers*
Berries (your choice, 1 cup whole)

DINNER

Calf's Liver Sautéed*
String Beans in Nutmeg Butter Sauce*

SNACK

Coconut meat

Week 2, Day 3 Recipes

CALF'S LIVER SAUTÉED

2 tablespoons butter
1 small onion, sliced
½ pound calf's liver, sliced
Sea salt to taste

Melt butter in a heavy skillet. Add onions and sauté until golden. Place liver pieces in the pan and cook until brown on both sides, turning once. Salt to taste.

COCONUT JUICE I

Liquid from 1 fresh coconut
Meat of ¼ fresh coconut

Place in a blender and blend until smooth.

FROZEN BANANA AND COCONUT

1 to 2 bananas
Enough grated coconut to cover

Roll bananas in coconut, pressing it into the banana. Wrap in tin foil and freeze—about 2 hours.

BANANA COCONUT SHERBET

1 recipe Coconut Juice (above)
1 ripe banana

Place ingredients in a blender and blend until smooth. Spoon into ice-cube trays and freeze. Stir sherbet once every hour until frozen—usually about 2 hours.

BUCKWHEAT AND PEPPERS

¾ cup water
½ teaspoon sea salt
¼ cup buckwheat, uncooked
2 green peppers, diced
¼ cup pine nuts

Bring the water and sea salt to a boil. Add the buckwheat. Lower heat and simmer, covered, for about 15 minutes. Add diced green peppers and cook 5 minutes more. Toss in pine nuts and serve.

STRING BEANS IN NUTMEG BUTTER SAUCE

1 cup whole fresh or frozen string beans
2 tablespoons butter
¼ teaspoon nutmeg, freshly grated or powdered
Sea salt to taste

Cook string beans. Melt butter, add nutmeg and salt. Pour on top of beans.

CHOPPED LIVER

2 tablespoons butter
¼ pound calf's liver, sliced
1 small onion, chopped
Sea salt to taste

Melt butter in a skillet and sauté liver until brown on both sides. Add onion and sauté 1 minute more. Remove contents of pan to chopping board or wooden chopping bowl and chop to relishlike consistency. Salt to taste.

E.E.'S STRING BEAN LOAF   Preheat oven to 325°

¼ cup buckwheat
1 teaspoon sea salt
½ sweet pepper, minced
1 small onion, minced
1 cup whole string beans, quartered

Bring ¾ cup water to a boil. Add buckwheat and salt. Reduce heat and simmer for 20 minutes (or until the water is absorbed). Remove to bowl. Steam peppers, onions, and string beans for 15 minutes. Add to the buckwheat and put into a loaf pan. Bake at 325° for 15 minutes.

WEEK 2, DAY 4

Foods Allowed for the Day

Duck, fresh or frozen, ½ medium, or substitute Cornish game hen or
    chicken
Broccoli or cauliflower, fresh or frozen, unlimited
Celery, unlimited
Pear, 2 fresh, or 4 slices dried
Currants, ¼ cup
Oranges, 2, or juice of 3
Cashews, up to ½ cup
Millet, ½ cup uncooked
Honey, up to 2 tablespoons
Cinnamon, unlimited
Beverage: mint tea

Suggested Menu Plan for the Day

BREAKFAST

Pear Bake*

LUNCH

Millet with Cashews and Cinnamon*

DINNER

Duck with Orange Sauce*
Steamed Broccoli

SNACK

Celery Sticks

Week 2, Day 4 Recipes

PEAR BAKE

1 fresh pear, cored and sliced
½ cup currants
2 slices dried pear

Place the dried pears in the bottom of a small glass casserole. Top with a layer of currants, a layer of fresh pears, and another layer of currants. Bake at 300° for ½ hour.

BROCCOLI SOUP

1 cup broccoli flowerets
2 stalks celery, minced
Sea salt
1½ cups water
⅛ cup millet, uncooked

Place the broccoli and celery in a saucepan and cover with water. Add ½ teaspoon salt. Cover pan and bring to a boil. Reduce heat and simmer for 25 minutes. Add millet and cook 20 minutes longer.

PEAR-CASHEW RELISH STICKS

2 slices dried pear
¼ cup cashews
⅛ teaspoon cinnamon
8 celery ribs

Chop pears and cashews to relish consistency. Season with cinnamon. Stuff into celery. Refrigerate.

MILLET WITH CASHEWS AND CINNAMON

½ cup millet
2 cups water, boiling
½ teaspoon sea salt
½ cup cashews
½ teaspoon cinnamon

Add millet to boiling salted water. Cook on a low heat for 15 minutes. Add cinnamon. Stir well and cook 15 minutes more. Mix in cashews. This makes at least 2 cups. For less food, cut recipe in half.

HONEY-GLAZED ORANGES

2 oranges, peeled and sectioned
2 tablespoons honey
⅛ cup water

Dip oranges in honey to coat them. Place coated oranges in a small baking dish. Sprinkle with water. Cover dish. Bake at 300° for 20 minutes.

STEWED PEARS AND CURRANTS

2 fresh pears, cored, peeled, and halved
¼ cup currants
2 tablespoons water

Place in a small saucepan. Simmer on low heat for ½ hour, stirring occasionally.

DUCK WITH ORANGE SAUCE   Preheat oven to 350°

Half of a 5-pound duck, fresh or frozen
Juice of 2 oranges
2 tablespoons honey

Place duck in a foil-lined roasting pan, cavity side down. If duck is frozen, be certain it has thawed completely. Prick skin of duck to release fat at least 3 times during baking. Roast at 350° for 45 minutes. Combine orange juice and honey. Mix well. Spoon over duck. Cook for ½ hour more, basting every 10 minutes.

COLD DUCK SALAD
(a summertime treat)

Half of a 5-pound duck
2 oranges, sectioned
¼ cup currants
½ teaspoon cinnamon

Roast duck at 350° for 1 hour and 15 minutes. Cool and refrigerate. Remove skin and discard. Remove meat, dice it, and place in a bowl with orange sections. Add currants. Sprinkle with cinnamon. Refrigerate for ½ hour.

WEEK 2, DAY 5

Foods Allowed for the Day

Scrod, fresh or frozen, or cod, unlimited
Potato, up to 2
Zucchini, fresh or frozen, or yellow squash, unlimited
Figs, fresh or dried, 4
Peaches, 2, or 4 slices dried
Walnuts, ½ cup, and 2 tablespoons walnut oil
Oats, ½ cup uncooked
Peanuts, ½ cup, and peanut oil, ½ cup used for frying only
Oregano, fresh or dried, unlimited
Ginger, fresh or dried, unlimited
Beverage: chamomile tea

Suggested Menu Plan for the Day

BREAKFAST

Oatmeal and Peaches*

LUNCH

Zucchini-Walnut Stir-fry*

DINNER

Codfish Cakes*
French Fried Potatoes*
Peanuts

SNACK

Figs

Week 2, Day 5 Recipes

OATMEAL AND PEACHES

4 dried peach slices, soaked in water, or 2 fresh peaches, sliced
1 serving oatmeal
Sea salt to taste

Dice peaches. Prepare oatmeal according to package directions. Mix peaches and oatmeal together.

OATMEAL BARS

½ cup peanuts
½ cup rolled oats, uncooked
8 figs chopped to size of currants

Place peanuts and oats in food processor or blender. Process. Add figs, process again (or chop all ingredients together until very fine). Press into 8-inch-square baking dish. Cover. Refrigerate for at least 2 hours. Cut into squares.

THE BEST FRENCH FRIED POTATOES

1 to 2 refrigerated, peeled potatoes, cut into finger-size pieces
½ cup peanut oil
Sea salt

Wash potatoes in cold water and dry well. Heat oil in a small deep pan until very hot. Put dry potatoes in the oil. Cook for 15 minutes. Remove potatoes, retaining oil in pan. Allow to drain on paper for ½ hour. Heat oil again and refry potatoes until golden brown. Salt to taste.

CODFISH CAKES

¼ pound frozen cod
1 medium-size potato, boiled
Peanut oil for frying

Wash fish well. Place fish in small pan. Cover with water. Bring water to boil and simmer for 10 minutes. Drain well. Mash potatoes in a bowl. Add codfish and mash again until well mixed. Heat the oil in a skillet. Drop cod mixture by the tablespoonful into the hot fat. Allow to brown on one side, turn, and brown the other side. Drain well on paper towel before eating.

ITALIAN PEANUTS

¼ cup peanuts
1 tablespoon peanut oil
¼ teaspoon dried oregano or ½ teaspoon fresh

Combine peanuts with oil. Place on baking sheet. Sprinkle with oregano. Bake in 300° oven for 10 minutes.

GINGERED WALNUTS

1 tablespoon walnut oil
⅛ teaspoon fresh ginger, minced
½ cup walnuts

Combine oil and ginger. Roll nuts in oil mixture. Place nuts on baking sheet and bake at 300° for 15 minutes.

ZUCCHINI-WALNUT STIR-FRY

1 to 2 zucchini, washed
1 to 2 tablespoons walnut oil
½ cup walnuts
⅛ teaspoon dried oregano (optional) or ¼ teaspoon fresh
Sea salt to taste

Slice zucchini into half-dollar-size pieces. Heat oil in heavy fry pan or wok. Add zucchini and stir-fry. Add walnuts and toss until they are warm. Sprinkle with oregano and salt and toss well.

BAKED SCROD IN FOIL

½ pound scrod
1 zucchini, sliced thin
¼ cup walnuts, shelled
1 tablespoon walnut oil
¼ teaspoon dried oregano or ½ teaspoon fresh
Sea salt to taste

Line a baking dish with foil. Place scrod on one-half of foil. Top with zucchini and walnuts. Sprinkle with walnut oil and oregano. Salt to taste. Bring other half of foil over the top and seal the edges. Prick holes in the foil with a fork. Bake at 325° for 25 minutes.

WEEK 2, DAY 6

Foods Allowed for the Day

Scallops, fresh or frozen, unlimited, or substitute turbot or mackerel
Mushrooms, fresh or frozen, 1 cup whole
Artichoke, fresh or frozen, unlimited, or asparagus, fresh or frozen, un-
    limited
Garlic, unlimited
Grapes, 1 cup whole, or ¼ cup white wine, used for cooking only
Pineapple, fresh, ½ small, or 4 slices dried, or 8 ounces of juice
Dates, 8
Chestnuts, 1 cup whole, or substitute water chestnuts
Olive oil, ¼ cup
Thyme, fresh or dried, unlimited
Beverage: comfrey tea

Suggested Menu Plan for the Day

BREAKFAST

Chestnuts and Dates*

LUNCH

½ fresh pineapple or 4 slices dried

DINNER

Garlic Asparagus Soup*
Scallopini with Mushrooms*
Steamed Artichoke*

SNACK

Grapes

Week 2, Day 6 Recipes

SCALLOP STEW

½ pound scallops
1 cup mushrooms, quartered
1 clove garlic, minced
¼ cup white wine
⅛ teaspoon thyme (optional)
Sea salt to taste

Place all ingredients in a small casserole. Cover and bake at 350° for 20 minutes or until scallops are cooked through.

SCALLOPINI WITH MUSHROOMS

2 tablespoons olive oil
1 clove garlic, minced
½ pound scallops, hammered thin
1 cup fresh mushrooms, quartered
Sea salt to taste

Heat oil in skillet. Add garlic and scallops. Sauté until brown. Add mushrooms and continue cooking until done (about 3 minutes). Salt to taste.

BAKED ARTICHOKE HEARTS

½ package frozen artichoke hearts, defrosted
1 cup mushrooms
1 clove garlic, crushed
pinch of thyme
2 tablespoons white wine
½ teaspoon sea salt

Place all ingredients in a small covered baking dish. Bake at 350° for 25 minutes.

STEAMED ARTICHOKE

1 large fresh artichoke
2 tablespoons olive oil
⅛ teaspoon minced garlic

Cut off stem of artichoke and trim off any bad leaves. Steam artichoke for 35 minutes. While it is steaming, heat oil and sauté garlic in it. Use garlic oil for dipping leaves.

MARINATED ARTICHOKE HEARTS   Must be prepared the night before.

1 package frozen artichoke hearts, defrosted
4 tablespoons olive oil (for marinating)
½ clove garlic
⅛ teaspoon dried thyme
¼ teaspoon sea salt

Mix oil, garlic, and thyme. Pour over artichokes. Refrigerate overnight.

GARLIC ASPARAGUS SOUP

4 garlic cloves, minced
½ quart boiling water
½ teaspoon sea salt
¼ teaspoon thyme
½ pound asparagus or 1 package frozen
1 tablespoon olive oil

Cook garlic, salt, and thyme in water for 20 minutes. Add asparagus and cook 20 minutes more. Place in blender and blend until smooth. Return to heat. Add olive oil in a slow, steady stream, beating constantly.

CHESTNUTS AND DATES

¾ cup chestnuts, roasted and shelled
8 dates

Chop dates and chestnuts together.

PINEAPPLE JAM DESSERT

1 cup pineapple, diced
8 dates, chopped
¾ cup shelled chestnuts, roasted (see p. 96)

Combine pineapple and dates in a small saucepan. Simmer gently for 20 minutes. Heat chestnuts in a 350° oven for 5 minutes. Top chestnuts with pineapple mixture.

WEEK 2, DAY 7

Special Test Day

Foods Allowed for the Day

Pork, ½ pound, boneless
Spinach, fresh or frozen, unlimited
Apples, 2 to 3
Spaghetti, 3 ounces
Butter, unlimited
Soy beans, ½ cup, 1 tablespoon soybean oil
½ loaf of It's Not Your Fault You're Fat Bread (recipe p. 129)

Today the following foods MUST be eaten at each meal:

BREAKFAST

2 to 3 apples

LUNCH

Spaghetti with butter sauce
½ loaf of It's Not Your Fault You're Fat Bread* with butter

DINNER

Broiled pork chops or pork roast
Steamed spinach

SNACK

Roasted Soybeans in Soy Oil*

Those who do not eat pork may choose a substitute from the "Eat Any-where" foods listed in Appendix E.

Special Test Day Recipes

IT'S NOT YOUR FAULT YOU'RE FAT BREAD

2 cups unbleached white flour
1 package yeast (1 tablespoon)
¾ to 1 cup whole-wheat flour (approx.)
½ tablespoon sugar
1 teaspoon salt
¼ teaspoon baking soda
1 cup milk
¼ cup water
Butter to grease pan

Warm mixing bowl in the oven. Combine white flour, yeast, sugar, salt, and soda in the bowl. Mix well. Heat liquids until very hot but not boiling. Add to dry ingredients. Beat well. Begin to add whole-wheat flour ½ cup at a time until dough begins to stiffen. Grease a small baking pan, place stiff dough in pan, cover, and set in the oven (which has been turned off) to rise for 1 hour. Remove cover and bake at 400° for 20 minutes (may need 5 minutes longer). Remove from oven, turn bread out of pan, and allow to cool on a rack.

ROASTED SOYBEANS IN SOY OIL   Preheat oven to 350°

½ cup soybeans
1 tablespoon soybean oil
Sea salt to taste

Combine soybeans and oil. Place in a baking dish, salt, and bake at 350° for 10 minutes.

WEEK 3, DAY 1

Foods Allowed for the Day

Clams or oysters, fresh or canned, unlimited
Tomatoes, fresh, 2, or 8-ounce can, or 8 ounces tomato juice
Avocado, ½, and 1 tablespoon avocado oil, and 1 bay leaf
Spaghetti squash, 1 to 2 pounds
Lemon, unlimited
Apricots, 4, or 8 dried
Sesame seeds or sesame oil, ¼ cup

Chives, fresh or dried, unlimited
Pecans, up to ½ cup halved
Hazelnuts, ½ cup whole
Beverage: ginseng tea

Suggested Menu Plan for the Day

BREAKFAST

Apricots and sesame seeds

LUNCH

Avocado-Hazelnut-Chive Salad*

DINNER

Clam Stew*
Baked Spaghetti Squash*

SNACK

Pecans

Week 3, Day 1 Recipes

AVOCADO AND APRICOT SALAD

½ avocado, peeled, pitted, and diced
8 dried apricots soaked in water for 1 hour
1 teaspoon sesame seeds
2 teaspoons lemon juice

Cut apricots in half. Toss with sesame seeds and avocado. Top with lemon juice and toss again.

GUACAMOLE

½ avocado, peeled
½ tomato, chopped fine
1 teaspoon chopped chives
Juice of ½ lemon
Sea salt to taste

Mash avocado. Mix all other ingredients together and blend with avocado.

AVOCADO-HAZELNUT-CHIVE SALAD

1 avocado, peeled
1 teaspoon chives, chopped
½ cup hazelnuts, chopped
Juice of ½ lemon
Sea salt

Mash avocado and chives together. Top with hazelnuts. Sprinkle with lemon juice and sea salt.

BAKED SPAGHETTI SQUASH

1 spaghetti squash, 1 to 2 pounds

Hammer 20 holes into the spaghetti squash with a long, heavy nail. Place in a preheated 350° oven for 45 minutes to 1 hour (until soft). Cut open, remove seeds, and scoop out "spaghetti" with a large spoon. Top with Clam Stew (recipe follows).

CLAM STEW

2 tomatoes, roughly chopped
20 cherrystone or littleneck fresh clams, shucked, or 1 can with broth
1 bay leaf
Sea salt to taste

Place ingredients in a small, heavy, covered saucepan. Bring to a boil, reduce heat, and simmer for 8 to 10 minutes. Serve on Baked Spaghetti Squash.

STEAMED CLAMS

20 steamer clams, or 1 can with broth
2 tablespoons avocado oil
Juice of ½ lemon
½ teaspoon sesame seeds

Thoroughly scrub clams. Place in a pot with ½ inch of salted water. Cover and steam for 6 to 10 minutes (until shells open). Heat avocado oil. Add lemon and sesame seeds. Dip clams into sauce.

SAUTÉED CLAMS AND TOMATOES

2 tablespoons avocado oil
20 fresh cherrystone clams, shucked, or 1 can with broth
2 fresh tomatoes, quartered
½ tablespoon fresh chives, chopped, or 1 teaspoon dried
Sea salt to taste

Heat oil. Add clams and tomatoes. Sauté. Sprinkle with chives and salt.
Mix well. Total cooking time should be about 6 to 8 minutes.

APRICOTS AND SESAME SEEDS SNACK

8 dried apricots
½ teaspoon sesame seeds
Juice of ½ lemon

Place apricots in small glass baking dish. Sprinkle with lemon juice and
sesame seeds. Bake at 300° for 15 minutes or until apricots give off their
juices.

WEEK 3, DAY 2

Foods Allowed for the Day

Lamb, fresh or frozen, ½ pound
Tuna (water-packed or fresh), unlimited
Carrots, 4
Cabbage, ½ small head
Kiwi fruit (Chinese gooseberries), 2
Strawberries, blackberries, or raspberries, fresh or frozen, unsweetened,
    1 cup whole
Macadamia nuts, ½ cup shelled, or substitute filberts
Coconut, ½ fresh or ¼ cup grated or 2 tablespoons dried
Brown rice, ½ cup uncooked
Peppermint, dried or fresh, unlimited
Beverage: peppermint tea

Suggested Menu Plan for the Day

BREAKFAST

Kiwi-Strawberry Ambrosia* with fresh mint

LUNCH

Tuna-Carrot Salad*

DINNER

Stuffed Cabbage with Lamb and Brown Rice*

SNACK

Macadamia Nuts

Week 3, Day 2 Recipes

FROSTY NUT SHAKE

1 recipe Coconut Juice II (p. 134)
3 ice cubes
½ cup macadamia nuts

Place ingredients in blender and blend until smooth and frosty.

KIWI-STRAWBERRY AMBROSIA

1 kiwi fruit, peeled and sliced
10 strawberries, halved
¼ cup fresh coconut, grated on large side of grater, or 2 tablespoons dried,
    unsweetened, grated coconut

Toss together.

PIÑA COLADA

1 recipe Coconut Juice II (p. 134)
¼ cup fresh grated coconut
1 kiwi fruit, quartered
3 ice cubes

Place in blender and blend until smooth.

COCONUT JUICE II

The liquid inside the coconut is ideal, but if you do not have it, you can make it. Use:

½ cup grated coconut, fresh or dried, unsweetened
½ cup boiling water

Put coconut in water and allow it to stand at room temperature for ½ hour. Place in the blender and blend until smooth.

LAMB-COCONUT PATTIES

½ pound ground lamb
2 tablespoons dried coconut, unsweetened
Sea salt to taste

Mix ingredients together. Shape into patties. Broil or charcoal-grill.

STUFFED CABBAGE WITH LAMB AND BROWN RICE

¼ cup brown rice
¾ cup water
½ pound lean lamb, ground
1 cabbage (approximately 1 pound)
2 tablespoons water
Sea salt to taste

Bring water to a boil. Add rice and simmer, covered, for 30 to 40 minutes. Mix rice, lamb, and salt. Blend well. Separate leaves of cabbage. Place leaves in saucepan and cover with water. Add ½ teaspoon sea salt. Bring water to a boil. Allow cabbage to boil for 5 minutes. Remove leaves from water without breaking them. Dry 4 of the largest leaves. Divide lamb into 4 patties. Place one patty on each of the 4 leaves and roll the leaves up. Shred the remaining leaves and place in the bottom of a heavy saucepan. Add ¼ cup of water and the cabbage rolls. Cover and simmer for 1 hour.

TUNA-CARROT SALAD

2 to 4 fresh carrots, scraped and grated
1 to 2 cans water-packed tuna, drained
Sea salt to taste

Flake tuna with a fork. Add grated carrots. Toss together. Add salt. Toss again.

BAKED FRESH TUNA, MACADAMIA   Preheat oven to 450°

½ cup macadamia nuts
1 pound fresh albacore tuna (1 inch thick)
Sea salt to taste

Put macadamia nuts in blender and blend until butterlike. Spread on fresh tuna. Bake at 450° for 15 minutes.

WEEK 3, DAY 3

Foods Allowed for the Day

Red snapper, fresh or frozen, unlimited, or substitute halibut, fresh or
    frozen (see fish-cooking directions in Appendix B).
Onion, 1 large
Peppers, sweet green or red, 2
Zucchini or yellow squash, fresh or frozen, unlimited
Yam or sweet potato, fresh or frozen, up to 2
Banana, 1 to 2
Oranges, 2, or 8 ounces juice
Currants, ¼ cup
Pine nuts, ¼ cup, or substitute peanuts
Safflower oil, ¼ cup
Beverage: papaya leaf tea

Suggested Menu Plan for the Day

BREAKFAST

Oranges and currants

LUNCH

Banana-Yam Mash*

DINNER

Broiled red snapper
Zucchini-Onion-Green Pepper Stir-fry*

SNACK

Pine nuts

Week 3, Day 3 Recipes

STEWED ONIONS AND CURRANTS

1 large onion, quartered
2 tablespoons currants
1 tablespoon water
1 slice orange peel

Put onion, currants, and water into a small, heavy saucepan. Top with orange peel (try to find an orange that has not been injected with red dye—one that is not bright orange). Cover pan and simmer very gently for 15 to 20 minutes or until onions are tender.

RED SNAPPER, ONION, AND PINE NUT BAKE

Safflower oil for greasing pan
½ pound red snapper, filleted
1 onion, sliced fine
2 tablespoons pine nuts
1 tablespoon safflower oil
Sea salt to taste

Place fish in a well-greased baking pan. Top with onion, pine nuts, safflower oil, and salt. Bake at 400° for 15 minutes. Turn on the broiler and broil for 1 minute.

ZUCCHINI-ONION-GREEN PEPPER STIR-FRY

½ fresh zucchini, sliced thin
2 tablespoons safflower oil
½ green pepper, sliced
1 small onion, sliced
1 tablespoon pine nuts
Sea salt to taste

Place 1 tablespoon safflower oil in a wok or heavy fry pan. Allow to get hot. Add zucchini, green peppers, and a pinch of sea salt. Stir-fry for 3 minutes. Remove and keep warm. Add rest of oil to wok, heat, and add onion and a pinch more of sea salt. Stir-fry for 3 minutes. Add pine nuts. Return zucchini and pepper to wok. Toss well. Stir-fry 1 minute more.

BAKED RED SNAPPER AND BANANAS   Preheat oven to 400°

Safflower oil for greasing
½ pound of red snapper, filleted
1 banana, halved lengthwise
Sea salt to taste

Grease a baking pan. Salt red snapper and place in baking pan. Lay banana halves on top. Brush with safflower oil. Bake for 15 to 20 minutes at 400° (until fish flakes).

BANANA-YAM MASH

1 yam
1 banana

Bake yam in a 450° oven for 1 hour. Split open and remove insides to a small bowl, reserving skin whole. Slice banana into bowl and mash banana and yam together. Return to shell. Place in 350° oven for 5 minutes.

VEGETABLE STEW

½ yam, sliced
½ green pepper, sliced
1 small zucchini, sliced
1 small onion, sliced
Sea salt to taste
¼ cup water

Place all ingredients in a small, heavy saucepan. Cover pan and simmer gently for 45 minutes or until vegetables are tender.

ORANGE AND CURRANT SWEET FISH   Preheat oven to 400°

Safflower oil to grease pan
½ pound red snapper, filleted
1 orange, peeled and in slices
Sea salt to taste
2 tablespoons currants

Grease baking pan. Place red snapper in pan. Top with oranges and currants. Bake at 400° for 15 to 20 minutes.

FROZEN BANANAS

1½ tablespoons pine nuts
1 banana

Roast pine nuts in 350° oven for 10 minutes. Peel banana. Roll banana in roasted pine nuts, pressing them in firmly. Wrap in plastic wrap and freeze.

WEEK 3, DAY 4

Foods Allowed for the Day

Turkey, fresh or frozen, or turkey parts, unlimited
Mushrooms, fresh or frozen, unlimited
Parsley, unlimited
Cherries, fresh or frozen, 1 cup whole
Wild rice, ½ cup cooked, or substitute oats
Plain yogurt, up to 8 ounces
Walnut oil or walnuts, ¼ cup
Honey, up to 2 tablespoons
Vanilla, unlimited
Thyme, fresh or dried, unlimited
Beverage: chamomile tea

Suggested Menu Plan for the Day

BREAKFAST

Vanilla Yogurt*

LUNCH

Wild Rice with Mushrooms and Thyme*

DINNER

Turkey Breast with Walnut Parsley Stuffing*

SNACK

Cherries

Week 3, Day 4 Recipes

TURKEY SOUP

2 cups Turkey Soup (p. 97)
1 cup leftover cooked turkey meat, defrosted and diced
6 mushrooms, sliced
1 teaspoon chopped parsley
⅛ teaspoon dried thyme or ¼ teaspoon fresh

Heat soup. Add mushrooms, parsley, and thyme. Simmer 10 minutes. Add turkey and simmer 3 minutes more.

VANILLA YOGURT

½ vanilla bean, or 1 teaspoon vanilla extract
1 cup plain yogurt (store-bought or homemade)
1 teaspoon honey (optional)

Split vanilla bean lengthwise. Scrape the insides into the yogurt and mix well. Refrigerate for ½ hour so the flavors will blend. Honey may be added for sweetness.

FROZEN YOGURT

2 cups plain yogurt
½ cup pitted cherries
2 tablespoons honey

Prepare yogurt the day before (or buy in the health-food store). Add cherries and honey. Mix well and place in the freezing compartment of an ice-cream maker. Churn until firm.

TURKEY BREAST WITH WALNUT PARSLEY STUFFING

Preheat oven to 350°

6 to 8 fresh parsley sprigs
½ cup shelled walnuts
1 large onion
Sea salt
1 small turkey breast

Chop walnuts and parsley together. Season with sea salt. Rub turkey breast with sea salt. Place onion-parsley mixture in the center of a baking dish. Top with turkey breast (meat side up). Bake at 350° for 20 minutes per pound.

WILD RICE WITH MUSHROOMS AND THYME

½ cup wild rice, uncooked
1½ cups water
1 cup whole mushrooms, washed
¼ teaspoon dried thyme or ½ teaspoon fresh thyme

Place rice in a pan. Cover with water. Bring to a boil, reduce heat, and simmer covered for 20 minutes. Add mushrooms and thyme and cook 10 minutes more until rice is soft.

PARSLEYED MUSHROOMS

1 cup whole mushrooms, washed
10 sprigs parsley, chopped
1 tablespoon walnut oil

Roll mushrooms in chopped parsley. Heat walnut oil until hot. Sauté mushrooms in hot oil for 5 minutes.

HONEY-GLAZED TOASTED WALNUTS   Preheat oven to 350°

½ cup shelled walnuts
2 tablespoons honey

Dip walnuts in honey. Place foil in a baking dish. Put walnuts on foil. Bake at 350° for 10 minutes.

CHERRY JAM

1 cup whole cherries, fresh or frozen
2 tablespoons water
1 tablespoon honey

Halve and pit cherries. Place in a small, heavy saucepan with 2 table-spoons of water. Simmer gently for 20 minutes. Remove from pan. Sweeten with honey. Mix well. Refrigerate.

WEEK 3, DAY 5

Foods Allowed for the Day

Swordfish or salmon, fresh, frozen, or canned, unlimited; or substitute bluefish (see fish-cooking instructions in Appendix B).

Bacon or ham, 5 slices (no nitrates when possible)
Garlic, unlimited
Asparagus, fresh or frozen, unlimited
Figs, 4
Almonds, ½ cup whole
Eggs, 3
Buckwheat, ½ cup uncooked
Olive oil, ¼ cup
Pumpkin seeds, ½ cup in shells
Beverage: comfrey tea

Suggested Menu Plan for the Day

BREAKFAST

Bacon and Egg Soufflé*

LUNCH

Buckwheat with Figs and Almonds*

DINNER

Swordfish with Garlic Oil*
Steamed asparagus with garlic

SNACK

Pumpkin seeds

Week 3, Day 5 Recipes

ASPARAGUS-BACON-EGG SALAD

½ pound asparagus, raw
5 slices bacon (no nitrates)
2 eggs, hard-boiled and shelled
Sea salt

Wash asparagus. Dry. Fry bacon and drain on paper towel. Chop bacon and hard-boiled eggs together. Steam asparagus. Top with bacon and egg mixture and serve.

SWORDFISH WITH GARLIC OIL   Preheat oven to 425°

½ pound swordfish, 1 inch thick
2 tablespoons olive oil
2 cloves garlic, minced
Sea salt to taste

Sauté garlic in hot oil for 1 minute. Place a sheet of foil in a baking pan. Place fish on foil. Add garlic-oil mixture. Wrap the foil around fish and seal edges. Bake at 425° for 25 minutes.

GARLIC ASPARAGUS EGG DROP SOUP

1 recipe Garlic Asparagus Soup (p. 127)
1 egg

Bring soup to a rolling boil. Beat egg. Dribble egg into soup very slowly. Mix with a fork. Serve immediately.

ROASTED PUMPKIN SEEDS   Preheat oven to 350°

2 tablespoons olive oil
½ cup pumpkin seeds
Sea salt

Spread olive oil on a baking sheet. Add pumpkin seeds and shake them around. Add salt. Bake at 350° for 5 minutes, shake again, and cook 3 to 5 minutes longer.

BACON AND EGG SOUFFLÉ   Preheat oven to 475°

1 small soufflé dish
6 slices bacon, cooked and well drained on paper towel
3 eggs
Sea salt

Place a waxed-paper cuff around the outside of soufflé dish (securing with string). Cook bacon until crisp. Use bacon fat to grease soufflé dish and inside of waxed-paper cuff. Separate eggs, being careful not to get any yolk in the whites. Beat yolks with ½ teaspoon bacon fat until smooth. Add a pinch of salt to whites and beat until stiff but not dry. Fold yolks and bacon into egg whites, being careful not to break down whites. Carefully transfer egg and bacon mixture to soufflé dish. This entire process is best done with a rubber spatula. Bake in 475° oven 10 minutes, lower heat to 400° and bake 20 minutes more. Soufflé is done when top is brown.

BACON ALMOND-BUTTER ROLLS

5 slices bacon
¼ cup almonds
Sea salt

Cook bacon halfway. Salt almonds and put through a food grinder or
process in a food processor or blender until of butterlike consistency. Refrigerate until firm. Place ½ teaspoon of almond butter at the end of each
bacon slice and roll up the slice. Refrigerate for ½ hour. Broil on the top
rack for 2 to 3 minutes.

BUCKWHEAT WITH GARLIC SAUCE

1½ cups water
½ teaspoon sea salt
½ cup buckwheat, uncooked
2 tablespoons olive oil
10 cloves garlic, mashed

Bring water and salt to a boil. Add the buckwheat, reduce heat, and simmer, uncovered, for about 20 minutes or until done. Bake garlic cloves at
350° in small baking dish for 25 minutes or until garlic is soft. Squeeze
garlic out of skin. Mash. Mix with buckwheat.

BUCKWHEAT WITH FIGS AND ALMONDS

1½ cups water
½ teaspoon sea salt
½ cup buckwheat
6 figs, fresh or dried, quartered
¼ cup almonds

Bring the water and salt to a boil. Add buckwheat, reduce heat, and simmer, covered, for about 20 minutes. Mix in figs and almonds. (This makes
about 2 cups. For less food, decrease recipe.)

WEEK 3, DAY 6

Foods Allowed for the Day

Beef, ½ pound
Sardines, canned, unlimited
Spinach, fresh or frozen, unlimited

Potato, up to 2
Dates, 8
Blueberries, fresh or frozen, unsweetened, 1 cup
Filberts, 1 cup whole
Matzoh (wheat, salt, and water—read label), 1 large cracker
Peanuts, ½ cup, or peanut oil, ¼ cup
Ginger, fresh or powdered, unlimited
Beverage: sassafras tea

Suggested Menu Plan for the Day

BREAKFAST

Peanut Butter* and Gingered Blueberry Jam* on matzoh

LUNCH

Filberts and dates

DINNER

Beef—½ pound steak
Baked potato with sea salt and beef juices
Steamed spinach

SNACK

Sardines

Week 3, Day 6 Recipes

SPINACH-POTATO PANCAKES

1 large potato, peeled and grated
½ pound spinach, fresh, trimmed
¼ teaspoon sea salt
¼ cup peanut oil for frying

Get as much moisture as possible out of the grated potato by placing it in a strainer and pressing liquid out. Chop spinach and mix with potato. Add salt. Heat oil in a small, heavy skillet until very hot. Fry potato mixture by tablespoonfuls, turning once to brown both sides.

PEANUT BUTTER

Sea salt
½ cup peanuts
1 teaspoon peanut oil

Salt nuts. Place in a blender with peanut oil and puree. Store covered in the refrigerator.

BAKED POTATO WITH TOASTED PEANUTS

1 large potato, baked
¼ cup peanuts
1 tablespoon peanut oil
Sea salt to taste

Mix peanuts with peanut oil and salt. Spread on a small baking sheet in 350° oven for 5 minutes. Remove from oven, chop, and place in bowl. Split potato and scoop insides into the bowl with peanuts. Mix well and return to potato shell. Reheat for 5 minutes at 350°.

BEEF STIR-FRY

2 tablespoons peanut oil
½ pound fresh spinach
¼ teaspoon fresh ginger, minced
½ pound steak, cut into finger-shaped pieces
Sea salt to taste

Heat 1 tablespoon of oil in a wok or heavy fry pan until very hot. Add spinach, ginger, and a pinch of salt. Stir-fry for 3 minutes, just until spinach begins to wilt. Remove to a platter and keep warm. Add other tablespoon of oil and the steak to wok. Sprinkle with salt. Stir-fry to desired doneness. Add cooked spinach, toss together, and serve.

GINGERED SPINACH WITH CHOPPED FILBERTS

½ pound fresh spinach
¼ teaspoon chopped ginger
¼ cup filberts
Sea salt to taste

Wash and dry spinach well. Place in a steamer. Top with ginger. Steam for 15 minutes. Roast filberts at 350° for 10 minutes. Chop filberts. Place spinach on a plate and top with chopped filberts.

GINGERED BLUEBERRY JAM

1 cup blueberries
¼ teaspoon ginger, peeled and minced

Place blueberries and ginger in a small, heavy saucepan. Cook over low heat for 20 minutes.

PEANUT-BUTTER BURGERS

½ pound ground beef
2 tablespoons Peanut Butter (p. 145)
½ teaspoon sea salt

Mix all ingredients together well. Shape into 2 burgers and broil.

GINGERED PEANUTS   Preheat oven to 350°

½ cup peanuts
1 tablespoon peanut oil
¼ teaspoon fresh ginger or ⅛ teaspoon ground dried ginger
¼ teaspoon sea salt

Mix peanuts and peanut oil together. Sprinkle with ginger and salt. Place on baking sheet and bake at 350° for 10 minutes.

WEEK 3, DAY 7

Special Test Day

Foods Allowed for the Day

Chicken, unlimited
Tunafish, fresh or canned in water
Kale, fresh or frozen, unlimited
Lettuce, unlimited
Peaches, 2
Oranges, 3
Sunflower oil, 2 tablespoons and sunflower seeds, ¼ cup
Cashews, ½ cup

Today the following foods MUST be eaten at each meal:

BREAKFAST

1 glass orange juice
2 oranges

LUNCH

Tuna with lettuce, sunflower oil, and toasted sunflower seeds

DINNER

Chicken and Kale Soup*
Broiled chicken with sea salt
4 slices dried peaches

SNACK

Cashews

Special Test Day Recipes

TOASTED SUNFLOWER SEEDS (FOR LETTUCE)   Preheat oven to 350°

½ cup sunflower seeds
1 tablespoon sunflower oil
Sea salt to taste

Combine ingredients in a small dish. Mix well. Place in a small baking dish and bake at 350° for 10 minutes. Remove seeds and oil from pan to put on lettuce.

CAROL GAUDREAULT'S CHICKEN AND KALE SOUP

1 3-pound chicken
1 box frozen kale or ½ pound fresh
Sea salt to taste

Simmer chicken in salted water to cover for 1 hour. Remove chicken from pot. Reserve 2 cups of stock for soup. Remove meat from chicken and freeze. Boil kale for 12 minutes. Place in a blender with ½ teaspoon sea salt. Blend. Add chicken stock to blender ½ cup at a time until 2 cups are blended in well. Reheat for 5 minutes.

Following you will find a summary of the foods allowed on each day of the It's Not Your Fault You're Fat Diet.

SUMMARY OF ALLOWED FOODS

Week 1

Day 1	Day 2	Day 3	Day 4	Day 5	Day 6	Day 7
Crab, unlimited, or substitute cod or scrod	Turkey, unlimited	Flounder, unlimited	Lamb, 1/2 pound	Scallops, unlimited, or substitute sole	Salmon or swordfish, unlimited, or substitute turbot	Beef, 1/2 pound
Avocado, 1 small	Broccoli, unlimited	Carrots, 3 large	Eggplant, 1 medium or 2 small	Mushrooms, unlimited	Spinach, unlimited	Figs, 4
Alfalfa sprouts, unlimited	Yam or sweet potatoes, up to 2	Onion, 1 large	Peaches, 2, or 4 slices dried	Pea pods, 1 cup	Brussels sprouts, unlimited	Watermelon or honeydew, unlimited
Cantaloupe, 1 small	Currants, 1/2 cup	Grapefruit, 1 medium, or 8 ounces grapefruit juice	Banana, 1 or 2	Avocado, 1 small	Bacon, nitrate free, 5 slices, and 1 tablespoon bacon fat	Potatoes, 1 to 2
Strawberries, blackberries, or raspberries, 1 cup whole	Prunes, 8	Dates, 8	Blueberries, 1 cup	Strawberries, blackberries, or raspberries, 1 cup whole	Apricots, 2 fresh, or 4 slices dried, and 1 tablespoon apricot oil	Corn (3 ears or unlimited kernels), corn oil (2 tablespoons), or popcorn (1/2 cup unpopped)
Pineapple, 1/2 small or 4 slices dried	Pears, 2, or 4 slices dried	Wild rice, 1/2 cup uncooked, or substitute oats	Walnuts, 1/2 cup shelled	Pineapple, 1/2 small, or 8 ounces pineapple juice, or 4 slices dried	Grapes, 1 cup, or raisins, 1/2 cup	Parsley, unlimited
Pecans, 1/2 cup, shelled	Chestnuts, 1 cup, whole, shelled	Peanuts, 1/4 cup, and 1 tablespoon peanut oil	Buckwheat, 1/2 cup uncooked	Cashews, 1/2 cup	Lemon, unlimited	Pecans, 1/2 cup shelled
Sesame seeds, unlimited, or 2 tablespoons sesame oil	Filberts, 1/2 cup, shelled	Water chestnuts, 1/2 cup slices	Olive oil, 1/4 cup, or 8 olives	Millet, 1/2 cup uncooked	Brazil nuts, 1/2 cup	Honey, 2 tablespoons
Rice cakes (rice and sea salt only), 4	Maple sugar or syrup, up to 2 tablespoons	Honey, up to 2 tablespoons	Cottage, farmer, or pot cheese, 1 cup	Safflower oil, 2 tablespoons	Eggs, 3	Beverage: any commercial tea
Mint leaves, unlimited	Nutmeg, unlimited	Tarragon, unlimited	Rosemary, unlimited	Ginger, unlimited	Pepper, unlimited	
Beverage: chamomile tea	Beverage: comfrey tea	Beverage: papaya leaf tea	Beverage: sassafras tea	Beverage: chamomile tea	Beverage: spearmint tea	

Week 2

Day 1	Day 2	Day 3	Day 4	Day 5	Day 6	Day 7
Shrimp, unlimited	Sole, unlimited	Calf or beef liver, unlimited, or substitute trout, and 2 tablespoons butter	Duck, 1/2 medium, or substitute Cornish game hen or chicken	Scrod or cod, unlimited	Scallops, unlimited, or substitute turbot or mackerel	Pork, 1/2 pound
Tuna, fresh, or canned in water	Lettuce, unlimited			Potato, up to 2		Spinach, unlimited
Peas, 1 cup	Cucumbers, 2		Broccoli or cauliflower, unlimited	Zucchini or yellow squash, unlimited	Artichoke, 2, or asparagus	Apples, 2 to 3
Tomatoes, 2, or 8 ounces sauce or juice	Radishes, unlimited	Onion, 1 large	Celery, unlimited	Figs, 4	Garlic, unlimited	Spaghetti, 3 ounces
Carrots, 3	Apples, 2, or 4 slices dried	String beans, unlimited	Pears, 2, or 4 slices dried	Peaches, 2, or 4 slices dried	Grapes, 1 cup whole	Butter
Papaya, 1, or 4 slices dried	Kiwi fruit (Chinese gooseberries), up to 2	Peppers, 2	Currants, 1/4 cup	Walnuts, 1/2 cup, and 2 tablespoons walnut oil	Pineapple, 1/2 small, or 4 slices dried	Soy beans, 1/2 cup, and 1 tablespoon soy oil
Blueberries, 1 cup	Almonds, 1/2 cup shelled, and 1 tablespoon almond oil	Bananas, 1 or 2	Oranges, 2, or juice of 3	Oats, 1/2 cup uncooked	Dates, 8	It's Not Your Fault You're Fat Bread (white flour, yeast, whole-wheat flour, sugar, salt, baking soda, milk, water, butter)
Macadamia nuts, 1/2 cup shelled, or substitute filberts	Brown rice, 1 cup uncooked	Strawberries, raspberries, or blackberries, 1 cup whole	Cashews, 1/2 cup	Peanuts, 1/2 cup, or 1/2 cup peanut oil	Chestnuts, 1 cup, or substitute water chestnuts	
Sesame oil, 1/4 cup, or seeds, 1/2 cup	Safflower oil, 1/4 cup	Pine nuts, 1/4 cup, or substitute hickory nuts	Millet, 1/2 cup uncooked	Oregano, unlimited	Olive oil, 1/4 cup	
Dill, unlimited	Vinegar, 1/4 cup	Coconut, 1/2 fresh or 1/4 cup grated or 2 tablespoons dried	Honey, up to 2 tablespoons	Ginger, unlimited	Thyme, unlimited	Beverage: rose hips tea
Beverage: ginseng tea	Beverage: comfrey tea	Buckwheat, 1/2 cup uncooked	Cinnamon, unlimited	Beverage: chamomile tea	Beverage: comfrey tea	
		Nutmeg, unlimited	Beverage: mint tea			
		Beverage: sassafras tea				

SUMMARY OF ALLOWED FOODS (*continued*)

Week 3

Day 1	Day 2	Day 3	Day 4	Day 5	Day 6	Day 7
Clams or oysters, unlimited	Lamb, 1/2 pound	Red snapper, unlimited, or substitute halibut	Turkey, unlimited	Swordfish or salmon, unlimited, or substitute bluefish	Beef, 1/2 pound	Chicken, unlimited
Tomatoes, 2, or 8 ounces tomato juice or sauce	Tuna, water packed or fresh, unlimited	Onion, 1 large	Mushrooms, unlimited	Bacon or ham, nitrate free, 5 slices	Sardines, unlimited	Tuna fish, fresh or water packed, unlimited
Avocado, 1/2, and 2 tablespoons avocado oil, 1 bay leaf	Carrots, 4	Peppers, 2	Parsley, unlimited	Garlic, unlimited	Spinach, unlimited	Kale, unlimited
Spaghetti squash, 1 to 2 pounds	Cabbage, 1/2 small	Zucchini or yellow squash, unlimited	Cherries, 1 cup	Figs, 4	Potato, up to 2	Lettuce, unlimited
Lemon, unlimited	Kiwi fruit (Chinese gooseberries), 2	Yam or sweet potato, up to 2	Wild rice, 1/2 cup uncooked, or substitute oats	Almonds, 1/2 cup	Dates, 8	Peaches, 2
Apricots, 4, or 8 dried	Strawberries, blackberries, or raspberries, 1 cup whole	Bananas, 1 to 2	Plain yogurt, 8 ounces	Eggs, 3	Blueberries, 1 cup	Oranges, 3
Sesame seeds or oil, 1/4 cup	Macadamia nuts, 1/2 cup, or substitute filberts	Oranges, 2, or 8 ounces juice	Walnut oil or walnuts, 1/4 cup	Buckwheat, 1/2 cup uncooked	Filberts, 1 cup	Sunflower oil, 2 tablespoons, and seeds, 1/4 cup
Chives, unlimited	Coconut, 1/2 cup grated or 1/4 cup or 2 tablespoons dried	Currants, 1/4 cup	Honey, up to 2 tablespoons	Olive oil, 1/4 cup	Matzoh, 1 cracker	Cashews, 1/2 cup
Pecans, 1/2 cup	Brown rice, 1/2 cup uncooked	Pine nuts, 1/4 cup, or substitute peanuts	Vanilla, unlimited	Pumpkin seeds, 1/2 cup, in shells	Peanuts, 1/2 cup, or peanut oil, 1/4 cup	Beverage: sassafras tea
Hazelnuts, 1/2 cup	Peppermint, unlimited	Safflower oil, 1/4 cup	Thyme, unlimited	Beverage: comfrey tea	Ginger, unlimited	
Beverage: ginseng tea	Beverage: peppermint tea	Beverage: papaya leaf tea	Beverage: chamomile tea		Beverage: rose hips tea	

9

EVERY MEAL'S A TEST MEAL: THE QUICK WEIGHT LOSS DIET

The diet presented in this chapter is not for everyone. It is for you if you want to lose weight very quickly, and it is for you if you find that you do not feel well after many meals on the It's Not Your Fault You're Fat Diet and want to know why. But you should consult with your doctor before beginning this diet.

Many of us would rather eat tasty gourmet meals. Many of us *can* eat them with satisfaction and comfort as we lose weight by properly following the It's Not Your Fault You're Fat Diet; but some will find that they are not losing weight as fast as possible—or that they are allergically sensitive to many or most of the foods on the diet. When you eat several foods at each meal and are reacting to them, you may be confused about which foods are causing you to react.

One of the major benefits of following the Rotary Diversified Diet is that it unmasks your previously unrecognized food allergies. When that happens, you may feel uncomfortable, at least until your addictions are broken. But if you are one of the people with many food allergies, the Every Meal's a Test Meal Diet will immediately help you identify and understand your allergies and lose weight.

A MORE LIMITED ROTARY DIVERSIFIED DIET

The basic principles of the It's Not Your Fault You're Fat Diet come from the Rotary Diversified Diet, and these same principles are at the heart of the Every Meal's a Test Meal self-diagnostic weight-loss diet. For the first three weeks of this diet, you are allowed only one food per meal—four different foods a day if you choose to have an evening snack. That's not as difficult as it sounds, because this diet automatically and effectively stops all of your addictive cravings.

BREAK ALLERGIC ADDICTIONS

For the first four days of the diet, as the foods you had been eating before you started the diet are working their way out of your system, you may become uncomfortable, feeling many of your old familiar aches and pains, and perhaps also feeling hungry. *These are withdrawal symptoms.*

These can be difficult days for some, but you can prepare for this by keeping the home remedies from chapter 7 on hand and using them when needed to clear your symptoms. After you stop withdrawing from your food addictions (around the fourth or fifth day of the diet), every meal becomes a single-food test that accurately identifies the foods you are allergic to. Not only will you know if you are allergic to a food, but, because each food stands alone, you will know exactly what symptoms the food causes you when you react to it. You will be able to determine which foods actually cause hunger or thirst, which ones stimulate cravings for specific foods, and which foods cause fluid retention. Many of your old familiar mental or physical discomforts will probably also appear. Fluid retention will be easily diagnosable by checking your scale twice daily for sudden weight gains or looking at your hands and feet or in the mirror.

HOW THE DIET WORKS

We have eliminated all of the common offenders in the first five days of the diet, so addictive cravings for most people's "favorite" foods (wheat, sugar, corn, beef, milk, chicken, eggs, potatoes, yeast, soy, tomatoes, chocolate, coffee) should disappear. Each of the foods in the diet is repeated at intervals of five days or longer. Foods that belong to the same food families are spaced at least two days apart, because foods in the same family have substances in common that can build up in the system and cause reactions. For example, solanine is a chemical that is present in all of the nightshade-family vegetables, including eggplant, tomatoes, peppers, and potatoes. Or think of the cooking odors that come from cabbage, brussels sprouts, broccoli, and cauliflower. Don't they all smell the same?

It is important that you understand the principles of a rotary diet so you will know exactly how to construct one that is tailor-made for your specific needs. We have included a chart to show you the food family that each food belongs to (see Appendix D), but for now, all you have to do is follow the diet just as it is printed, eating one food at each of the three meals, with or without the snack. We have given you several foods to choose from at each meal, but you are to eat only one of them. We want you to have a choice so you can eat what you like best. If you find you are allergic to a food and have to delete it from your diet, we have made sure that you will have other foods to choose from at that meal. Finally, we have provided enough foods so you will be able to choose two per meal from the list after the first three weeks.

EVERY MEAL'S A TEST MEAL DIET USED FOR QUICK WEIGHT LOSS

Even if you do not believe that you are allergic to foods, this can be the diet for you if you wish to lose weight as quickly as possible. It is difficult to overeat when you are eating just one food per meal. After all, how many apples or string beans can you eat at one time—even if you eat for a full twenty minutes?

You will also find this diet convenient if you work and want to take your lunch with you each day. There are always at least one or two easily transportable foods listed for the day. At first, some of our patients feel hungry on this diet—but many do not. Whether or not you feel some hunger for a few days doesn't matter, because almost everyone feels so much better on it that they have no wish to go back to the way they felt before they began the diet.

Keep in mind that if you start your weight-loss program with this diet and find that you require more diversity in your foods, you can always switch to the two- and three-food meals of our It's Not Your Fault You're Fat Diet. It would be wise to complete the first six days of this diet and see how you feel on the evening of the sixth day before you make the change. Chances are that you will feel so well on this diet that you will want to stay on it for a good long time. You may do so for as long as you wish.

RULES FOR THE EVERY MEAL'S A TEST MEAL DIET

Rule 1: **No alcoholic beverages are to be consumed; smoking is highly undesirable; and chemical exposures are to be avoided.**

Rule 2:   **Follow the diet as printed. Choose one food for each meal from among the foods listed for each day, including at least one protein and one vegetable or fruit.**

Never eat the same food more than once a day. The fourth meal or evening snack is optional. Eat it only if you are hungry.

Rule 3:   **Allow your "Eating Habits Inventory" (chapter 5) to be your guide.**

When a day offers you a food that you love, crave, or eat frequently, include it in your day's eating. By testing food suspects one at a time, you will see what they really do to you. But avoid these foods during the first four days of the diet as these are your withdrawal days and the withdrawal symptoms, rather than the suspect food, could be causing your uncomfortable feelings.

Rule 4:   **Single-food meals should be eaten at least four hours apart until you have established which foods caused reactions.**

At the beginning, you probably will need more food to satisfy your appetite (usually about two to three times the amount you would ordinarily eat of that food). Relax when you eat, and chew your food thoroughly. Don't stuff yourself—eat just enough to take away your appetite. *Never eat for more than twenty minutes.*

If you are on this diet to test for allergies, the quantity of food you eat may be important. If you eat a large portion, you may have a reaction because a large amount of food allergen might be more than your body can tolerate. If this should happen, eat a smaller portion of the food the next time it appears on the diet, and see what happens.

Rule 5:   **Plan ahead.**

You should shop twice a week so you always have the fresh foods you need in the house and available for each meal. Many people take the diet with them when they go shopping to see which choices are available, fresh, and economically priced. Be sure to buy enough so you will not be hungry. You can always freeze leftovers or share them with other family members.

Rule 6:   **Sea salt is permitted.**

Lightly salt your food to taste. Avoid excess. If you are on a salt-restricted diet, do not use more than you are allowed. During the first three weeks, sea salt is the only seasoning permitted. In week four, you may begin to use the spices listed in the "miscellaneous" column.

Sea salt is made from evaporated seawater and may be purchased in your health-food store and some supermarkets. Kosher salt or sodium chloride (USP) also may be used, but they do not have all the minerals present in sea salt. Regular table salt often contains corn sugar (dextrose) or other added chemicals and should not be used.

Rule 7: **Buy fresh foods whenever possible.**

Frozen foods and foods canned in glass are also acceptable. Avoid foods in metal cans as much as possible; buy them only when there is nothing else available, as is usually the case with tuna or sardines. Read labels carefully and do not buy any foods that list additives, chemicals, stabilizers, sweeteners, artificial color or flavors, spices, or additional foods. (For example, buy tuna packed in water, not in oil.) If they are available to you, foods you are sure are organically grown are best.

Rule 8: **Foods may be prepared by being washed and eaten raw, dried (be sure to buy unsulfured dried fruits without preservatives), baked, broiled, boiled, steamed, or as a juice.**

You may not fry foods for the first three weeks because that would require an oil, which would be a second food.

Whenever possible, eat vegetables and fruits raw or lightly steamed to preserve their vitamins and enzymes. Juices are best consumed immediately upon being made. If you use juice concentrates, buy only the unsweetened kind, mix with spring water, and store in glass containers.

Avoid aluminum and nonstick cookware. Cook in Pyrex, Corningware, cast iron, stainless steel, or enamel cookware. (See cooking instructions in Appendixes A and B.)

Rule 9: **You may drink as much bottled spring water or untreated well water as you wish.**

Glass bottles are preferred over plastic containers, which often contaminate the water they hold. If you must drink chlorine-treated tap water, process it through a charcoal filter to remove the chlorine, or boil it for ten minutes, or you can place it in an open jar and expose it to the air for three days. Of course, you should always store it in glass bottles.

Rule 10: **Establish a food diary.**

If you react to a food, note this in your diary. Describe all of the resulting symptoms and their severity. If your reaction is very severe, do not test the food again for at least two or three months. If there is only a mild reaction to a food, test it again in five to seven days. It would be a shame to lose a "safe" food because of an error.

Rule 11:   During the first week, weigh yourself twice a day—in the morning after bladder and bowel elimination, and in the evening before going to bed.

There should not be more than a 2-pound net gain for the day. If you have gained more than 2 pounds during the day or fail to lose weight overnight, you are probably retaining water. If you can tell which food caused you to retain water, record that in your food diary as a severe reaction. (See Appendix C for a sample food diary page.) If you don't know the food, pay careful attention to each of the foods for that day the next time you eat them. Weigh yourself before and after you eat them and pay attention to any body puffiness that may be associated with that food.

Identifying the foods that cause you to retain water and eliminating them from your diet will make diuretics ("water pills") a thing of the past—positive proof that the doctor who prescribed this medication didn't realize that food allergy was causing your fluid retention.

After the first week, weigh yourself once a day just to follow your overall progress and alert you to the onset of any problems.

Rule 12:   You may eat your four foods in any order during the day, but choose from a variety of food groups.

You might choose a fruit or cereal for breakfast, a vegetable for lunch, meat or fish for dinner, and seeds or nuts for an evening snack. Or, for the sake of convenience, you can vary that order. This will make it simple for you to plan your meals to fit your schedule. It is easy to carry some raw vegetables, fresh fruit, nuts or seeds to work or school for lunch, or just to get a broiled chop or fillet of fish at a nearby restaurant.

A very few people may have severe allergic reactions to so many foods that they will have to substitute for the choices given. If you have reacted to most of the foods listed for a particular day, you must find some new foods to replace the offenders. To select your new foods, use the following simple rules.

RULES FOR SUBSTITUTION OF FOODS

Rule 1: **You may not repeat a food in your diet until at least four days have gone by since that food was eaten.**

This means if you eat peanuts on Monday, you may not have peanuts, organic peanut butter (without additives), or peanut oil until Friday. If you eat apples on Tuesday, you may not have apples, applesauce, apple juice, or dried apples until Saturday.

Rule 2: **Foods in the same family (see Appendix D) may not be eaten more often than once every other day.**

Food-family members are rotated on a two-day basis. Therefore, if you eat oranges or drink orange juice on Monday, you may not have grapefruit, lemons, or limes until Wednesday, because each of these fruits is a member of the citrus family. You must rotate foods in the same family every two days, and remember that the individual foods must not be repeated for at least four days. If you were rotating the citrus and apple family, it might look like this:

Monday	Tuesday	Wednesday	Thursday	Friday	Saturday	Sunday
Oranges	Apple	Grapefruit	Pear	Oranges	Apple	Grapefruit
or	or	or		or	or	or
Orange Juice	Apple Juice	Grapefruit Juice		Orange Juice	Apple Juice	Grapefruit Juice

Rule 3: **There is one further complication in formulating your rotary diet. Meals of "allergically identical" foods must be separated from each other by four days.**

When you review the food families in Appendix D, you will find that foods in some families are bracketed together. This is because some foods are so closely related (in the allergic sense) that they are almost identical. We treat these foods as if they were variations of one food. You may substitute any one of them for any other member of their group, but you must allow four days to elapse before eating any one of them again. A good example of this very close relationship is found in the grass family, among some cereal grains. Wheat, rye, barley, malt, and triticale (a hybrid of wheat and rye) are so closely related that they must be treated as one food. If you ate any of these grains on Monday, you could not eat another grain in this very closely related group until Friday.

**Rule 4:   The "Eat Anywhere" foods listed in Appendix E are not re-
lated to any other foods.**

They are "only children." There are no other family members
that require a two-day rotation with them. You may place them
anywhere in your diet as long as you eat any food in this group
only once every four days.

· Now that you know the rules, it is time to get started on the Every
Meal's a Test Meal–Quick Weight Loss Diet. Follow it and become thin
and allergy-free.

NOTES

1. Horizontal arrows placed to the right or left of a food indicate
that you may eat that food once—on *one* of the several consecutive days
indicated—during a given rotation cycle. The spacing intervals of five
days or more between ingestions of certain foods in this rotary diet provide a built-in broad flexibility of menu selection for you.

2. Slanted lines (/) between two or more foods indicate that, until
proven otherwise, these foods are to be treated in your diet plan as if they
are allergically "identical." They may be substituted for each other and
they must be rotated at four- to seven- day intervals with respect to each
other.

3. Foods that are enclosed in a bracket are members of the same
food family and they are to be rotated on at least a two-day basis. Foods
marked with an asterisk are also members of the same family and are to
be rotated on at least a two-day basis. The asterisk is used when a bracket
would not be suitable. (For example, on Day 3 of Week 1, apricots and
almonds are members of the same food family but apricots are listed in
the Fruit category and almonds in the Nuts category.)

4. Make a daily selection of three foods from different families for
your morning, noon, and evening single-food meals for at least the first
three weeks of your diet. An evening snack may be chosen from the foods
permitted for the day if you wish to eat a fourth food. *One of your daily
selections must be an 8- to 12-ounce serving of a high-protein food.* If
you want to lose weight even faster, you may eat two foods a day on a
regular basis for the first ten days of your diet, and for three- to five- day
periods every two weeks, being guided by your appetite and your pace of
weight loss.

EXAMPLE:

	Week 1, Day 1		Week 1, Day 5
	Honeydew		Oats
	Asparagus	3 foods	Artichoke
	Red Snapper		Chicken
		or	
	Plum		Pineapple
	Butterfish	2 foods	Turkey

5. Brown rice may be eaten in the form of cooked grain, plain rice cakes with or without salt, or puffed rice with nothing, no milk or sugar.

6. Sweeten cranberries, cranberry juice, or rhubarb with maple sugar, maple syrup, or honey, not cane sugar.

7. When milk is listed, cottage cheese, butter, unflavored yogurt, mozzarella cheese, farmer cheese, or ricotta cheese may be tested.

8. Oats may be eaten in the form of oatmeal, or puffed or shredded oats with no preservatives or other food additives.

WEEK 1

	Day 1	Day 2	Day 3	Day 4	Day 5	Day 6	Day 7
FRUIT / CEREALS	* { brown rice / wild rice } honeydew watermelon currant prune / plum	lime fig mango coconut	buckwheat *apricot { cranberry (or juice) blueberry }	millet grapefruit (or juice) persimmon pomegranate pear	currants pineapple cantaloupe* papaya	oats **tangerine date banana grape / raisin strawberry (or strawberry leaf tea)	*buckwheat nectarine plum / prune *rhubarb fig
VEGETABLES	asparagus sweet potato celery	spinach { turnip radish lentils black-eyed peas *bamboo shoots }	summer squash / zucchini avocado water chestnut onion eggplant	swiss chard / beet { carrot anise broccoli / cabbage mung bean sprouts } carob olive (or oil)	artichoke yam cucumber* potato	{ snow peas green peas soy tofu or oil celery parsnip parsley } watercress mushroom	spinach onion water chestnut avocado pumpkin (or seeds) acorn squash
PROTEIN	cod (scrod)→ red snapper→ butterfish shrimp chicken clams lamb	cod (scrod)→ red snapper→ scallops smelt sole	turkey→ mackerel lobster turbot	turkey→ crab→ chicken→ pork→ pink perch bass swordfish	turkey→ crab→ chicken pork→ milk sardines oysters	red snapper→ crab→ scallops→ pork→ shrimp sole haddock pickerel	red snapper→ crab→ scallops lobster→ beef / lamb→ tuna pompano porgy carp eggs
MISC. NUTS	sunflower seeds (or oil) filbert pine nut peppermint or lime mint tea	chestnut macadamia nut sassafras tea	sesame seeds or tahini *almond (or almond oil) real maple syrup nutmeg marjoram	Brazil nut black pepper thyme comfrey tea	walnut (or oil) pistachio { chives garlic spearmint tea }	chestnut *dill **lemon ginger	sesame seeds (or tahini or oil) honey peppermint tea

WEEK 2

	Day 1	Day 2	Day 3	Day 4	Day 5	Day 6	Day 7
CEREALS	brown rice		corn (or corn oil)	buckwheat	brown rice oats		molasses / cane sugar wild rice
FRUIT	apple	papaya apricot cherry pineapple lime	grape / raisin pear banana currants grapefruit	coconut peach plum / prune cantaloupe raspberry blackberry lemon	apple→ fig	orange→ apple mango *watermelon strawberry	currant papaya banana grape
VEGETABLES	kale / cauliflower / cabbage / brussels sprouts tomato oregano lettuce safflower oil carrot *chick pea	asparagus beet cucumber olive oil	green pepper eggplant string beans kidney beans lima beans artichoke rutabaga mustard greens or seed celery	yam scallion leeks swiss chard celery	potato→ lettuce cabbage / brussels sprouts / cauliflower / broccoli carrot *peas	potato→ *squash / yellow / zucchini / spaghetti squash onion celeriac spinach	water chestnut sunflower seeds turnip horseradish Chinese cabbage string beans alfalfa sprouts lima beans celery
PROTEIN	red snapper cod (scrod) shad lobster beef / lamb flounder	turkey ocean perch smelt	chicken herring turbot milk pork shrimp	sole haddock clams crab scallops	whitefish tuna silver perch eggs beef / lamb red snapper lobster	flounder tomcod turkey bass mackerel	pork→ milk→ shrimp→ chicken halibut trout
NUTS	cashew	*almond	pecan pistachio nut	chestnut	Brazil nut *soy nuts / tofu peanut	almond	pecan
MISC.	licorice tea fenugreek tea	rosemary thyme rose hip tea	sassafras tea	sarsaparila tea	spearmint tea honey	juniper tea	*licorice tea fenugreek tea

WEEK 3

	Day 1	Day 2	Day 3	Day 4	Day 5	Day 6	Day 7
CEREALS	buckwheat→	→buckwheat	brown rice corn		millet wheat/barley	buckwheat	oats corn
FRUIT	nectarine plum date pear blueberry	pineapple strawberry *honeydew	apple mango grape/raisin	banana grapefruit grapes/raisins currants *papaya	fig pear *raspberry	cherry apricot pineapple orange	grape/raisin mango apple *strawberry date
VEGETABLES	olive (or oil) tomato green pepper swiss chard beet	lentils→ peas→ carrots *cucumber **lettuce	→lentils →peas potato broccoli/brussels sprouts/cauliflower spinach onion	celery parsnip fennel zucchini endive escarole sweet potato	tomato eggplant string bean soy lima bean beet/swiss chard olive (or oil) rutabaga turnip kohlrabi	anise carrot water chestnut lettuce cucumber butternut squash	mustard greens cabbage/broccoli mung sprouts peas green pepper potato
PROTEIN	pork→ milk→ shrimp→ crab→ cod (scrod) swordfish scallops sole	red snapper→ milk eggs crab→ haddock whiting lobster	→red snapper→ tuna flounder →crab	→red snapper→ lamb/beef bluefish mackerel cod (scrod)	pork→ scallops smelt sole pink perch duck	pork→ eggs milk turkey haddock salmon lobster	→pork crab flounder trout whiting
NUTS	cashew	filberts sesame	walnut (or oil)	Brazil nut	cashew chestnut	sesame pecan	**peanut
MISC.	chestnut oregano	**comfrey tea	ginseng tea	honey *papaya leaf tea mint tea	garlic *raspberry leaf tea	cinnamon tea	*strawberry leaf tea

Congratulations. You have completed three weeks of the Every Meal's a Test Meal Diet. We are sure that you have learned a great deal about how your body works, have experienced a decrease in your appetite, and are losing weight.

By now you should have eliminated your food-allergy-driven compulsive-addictive eating patterns. You should also know which foods are causing your allergies. If you feel well at this phase of the diet, you may proceed in one of three ways.

1. After completing Week 3, you may repeat the three-week elimination rotary diet as many times as you wish. Go back to Week 1, Day 1, and rotate through again, trying additional foods, this time substituting them in place of some of the foods you ate during the first 21 days.

2. If you desire more variety and would like to eat more than one food per meal, you may choose two or three already tested foods from the lists offered for each meal. If you react to a combination of safe foods, note that in your food diary. Occasionally people are sensitive to a combination of foods although they can tolerate each food when it is eaten alone.

3. You may choose to go on the It's Not Your Fault You're Fat Diet, substituting foods from the "Eat Anywhere" list or the "Food Family Chart" for foods that caused you to have a severe reaction, according to the rules for substitution. You will continue to lose weight on any of the diets. Just remember that the less you eat, the more you lose. That is a fat and calorie fact of life.

Those of you who are ill as you follow the Every Meal's a Test Meal Diet really have an important allergic-ecologic health problem. If the food addictions that caused you to eat compulsively are gone and you still do not feel well, you may be sensitive to chemicals and airborne allergens as well as to the foods you have brought under control with this diet.

If you are allergic to chemicals and airborne allergens, you will need a physician qualified in the practice of clinical ecology to help you become well again. Finding a clinical ecologist may not be easy. There are many of them, however, and if you write to us,[1] or to the Society for Clinical Ecology, the secretary will be happy to send you a list of the clinical ecologists practicing in your part of the country. Mail your inquiries to: Dr. Del Stigler, 2005 Franklin, Suite 490, Denver 80205. Be sure to include a self-addressed stamped envelope.

Finding that you are allergic should not cause you to be discouraged about your diet or what may seem to be overwhelming difficulties that you are temporarily faced with. Be happy that you have found out what

[1] 3 Brush Street, Norwalk, CT 06850

has been causing your health problems and do something about it immediately. Do not go off of the diet! Do go to a qualified physician and find
out what other things you can do to bring your body to a state of optimal
health.

10

MAINTENANCE

Maintenance is the most important part of any diet. If you lose weight only to gain it back, the satisfaction and health benefits become very short-lived.

On our diet, maintenance is especially important. If you have done well on our diet—both lost weight and felt better—then you have established the fact that you have controlled an important allergy problem. You were allergically addicted to food, and as soon as you go off your diet, your allergic-addictive patterns will return.

The diets in this book cause you to think about what you eat, to plan your meals. When we don't plan our meals, we tend to eat what is available, and what we view as "available" are usually all our old favorites.

It is very easy to fall back into old eating patterns, but don't. It will not be good for your waistline or your health. What you must do is plan a rotation diet you can live on. Decide which foods you want to eat, and create a thoroughly satisfying one-week diet using those foods in rotation. Make sure that you eat each food only once every four days; foods in the same food family once every two to three days (see rotary diet rules on pp. 87–91).

By working out a one-week diet, you will have the same foods on the same day every week. You will be able to plan meals at home and meals eaten out. The foods for each day will become a part of your life— a healthy habit. We try to live this way, and find it a very easy way of life. There is never a question about what to have for dinner. Of course, I always try new combinations of foods and new ways to cook old favorites. You would be surprised at the endless variety of delicious meals possible on the maintenance diet.

We have designed a maintenance diet for you. Each day has at least twenty-five foods to choose from and many wonderful food-combination possibilities. Many of the days are similar to the It's Not Your Fault You're Fat Diet, and you will be able to use many of the recipes from that diet.

Consider each day a challenge and put on your creative-cook thinking caps. Fran would love to exchange recipes with you.

7-DAY MAINTENANCE DIET

Monday	Tuesday	Wednesday	Thursday	Friday	Saturday	Sunday
shrimp	pork	chicken	sole	beef	turkey	lobster
scallops	bacon	clams	turbot	veal	egg (chicken)	flounder
	ham			lamb		halibut
oyster	liver, beef or	cornish hen	pompano	chicken liver	red snapper	bass
	calf's					grouper
mussel		salmon	crab	herring	tuna	pickerel
	scrod (cod)	trout		shad	mackerel	northern pike
snail	haddock		broccoli			
duck	pollack fish	caviar	cauliflower	celery	carp	butter
		sturgeon	cabbage	dill/fennel		cheese
			brussels sprouts		yam	milk
pike	garlic	soy bean/tofu	radish	chives	lettuce	green pepper
	asparagus	lima bean	turnip	scallion	chickory	eggplant
tilefish		alfalfa sprouts		onion	endive	
	carrot	lentils	buckwheat	leek	escarole	rutabaga
dolphin fish	cumin/coriander					
			peach	swiss chard	romaine	wheat, rye,
ocean perch	okra	mushroom	plum (prune)	beets		barley, millet,
					cucumber	triticale
sweet pea	fig	acorn squash	orange	navy bean	yellow squash	
blackeyed pea		butternut squash	lemon	kidney bean	spaghetti squash	yeast
chick pea	peach	hubbard squash		string bean	zucchini	
(garbanzo)			chestnuts			
split pea	pineapple	bamboo shoots	pistachio nuts	mung bean sprouts	pumpkin	grapefruit

pea pods, snow	persimmon	oats/wild rice	sesame seeds	potato	watermelon	lime
spinach	mango	date	sesame oil	corn	blueberry	banana
avocado	cashew	strawberry	artichoke	rice, brown	cranberry	plantain
currant	sweet potato	raspberry	safflower oil	grape	apricot	rhubarb
Spanish melon	maple syrup	blackberry	sorrel	(raisin)	almond	lichee nut
cantaloupe	maple sugar	apple	thyme	papaya	almond oil	black pepper
casaba melon	mustard greens	hazelnut	sage	kiwi fruit	cherry	watercress
cranshaw melon	olive	Chinese water-	rosemary	coconut	nectarine	horseradish
Persian melon	olive oil	chestnut	allspice	pine nut	pumpkin seeds	chocolate
honeydew	nutmeg	walnut		cinnamon	basil	caraway
pear	clove	walnut oil		pecan	marjoram	parsley
macadamia nut		ginger		peanut	mint	parsnip
Brazil nut		turmeric		peanut oil	tarragon	hickory nut
sunflower		cardamom				
oil		bay leaf				
seeds		paprika				
filbert		chili powder				
saffron		tomato				
oregano		cayenne				
savory						

Horizontal lines separate food families.
Brackets indicate the enclosed foods are allergically "identical."

There are a few suggestions we would like to make based on our experience on the diet.

If there is a food listed that you know will cause uncomfortable symptoms or affect your appetite or your weight (retain water), don't include it in your diet until you have tested it and find that you are no longer bothered by it.

When there is a special occasion (try not to make it more than once a week) and you go off the diet, you may have some symptoms, but you probably have not done much damage. Go back on the diet for the very next meal as if you had not gone off it at all, but reduce the portions of those foods that you "cheated on."

Make it a habit to carry a little notebook with each day's foods noted in it. I also keep a list of the day's foods and the recipes on the kitchen counter, as a reminder both for shopping and for eating. It works like a charm—like an old friend helping me to stay on course.

If I do eat something that is not listed on the diet for the day, I never feel guilty. This is not a guilt-provoking eating plan. If you go off it once in a while, nothing serious should happen (unless you are severely allergic to the food you eat). Your problems will begin again if you continue to eat the same foods too often, day after day. If you carelessly overload your system, food addiction will creep up on you. Marshall always warns his patients, "Once a food addict, always a food addict." Re-addiction is a very subtle process that gradually catches up with the delinquent dieter.

Keep in mind that you cannot stop reading labels on foods. It is easy to become lax and buy prepared foods that are complex mixtures that frequently contain hidden foods, and some of the ingredients are not printed on the labels. Be careful of that. Continue to buy fresh foods. They are so much healthier for you and your family. Both of our diets are exceptional not only as weight-loss diets, but as health tools. They can, if you allow them to, be the cornerstone of your health, improving the quality of your life immeasurably.

Most important: If you gain 2 or 3 pounds and keep them for three days or longer, begin the diet you lost your weight on again from Day 1. You will probably lose the unwanted pounds by the end of the first week, and you may find out what foods caused the weight to come back on.

On our diet, you will gain new insight into your old eating habits. You will learn which foods to stay away from because they make you eat compulsively, or retain water, or give you some other reaction. You will probably feel and look better than you have in years. Remember how you feel and look. Do your best to stay that way. It is one of the most important things you will ever do for yourself and those who care about you.

11

TIPS

The tips in the following pages are the results of many people's experiences. Marshall's patients share them with you, and they, as we, hope your days on the diet will be made easier and more fun because of them.

SETTING GOALS

Before you start one of our diets, take some time to consider the reasons why you are going on the diet.

Ask yourself: How much weight do I want to lose?

Picture yourself as you want to look, and keep that ultimate goal in your mind.

What are your health goals? Do you want to breathe easier? feel more energetic? lower your blood pressure?

Goals help you stay on a diet, so keep them in mind at all times.

PLANNING

1. On our diet, you must *plan ahead*. Decide if you want to go on the It's Not Your Fault You're Fat Diet or the Every Meal's a Test Meal Diet.
2. Think through your week to see how the diet will fit into your plans.
3. Decide which time of the day is best for you to have your main hot meal. Some people like more food at lunch than at dinner. You decide. If you want to, there is no reason not to have meat (or poultry or fish) and vegetables for breakfast.
4. Buy a pocket-size notebook or daily log to be used as a "food diary."

Carry it with you and record your reactions to foods, and environmental factors if you suspect chemicals, pollens, dust, or molds are bothering you. (See food diary sample page in Appendix C.)

5. If there are some foods you look forward to more than others, save them for the evening. In the beginning, it's often easier to get through the day if you know there is a "reward" waiting.

6. When you are going to be away from home, make sure you carry with you all of the foods you will need for the day so you won't become too hungry and be tempted to go off your diet.

7. Try to locate at least one restaurant near your place of work that will cook your food exactly as you ask. Restaurants usually add a number of ingredients even to simple dishes.

8. Carry a Thermos or large glass bottle of spring water or dechlorinated tap water with you—or plan to drink mineral water, seltzer, or club soda. Seltzer and club soda are manufactured chlorine-free because chlorine would cause an unpleasant taste in the alcoholic beverages with which they often are mixed.

9. Begin the It's Not Your Fault You're Fat Diet on a day that will make your test day (Day 7) the most convenient day for you not to feel so great if you should have any food reactions. If Sunday will be the most convenient day to rest, then begin the diet on Monday.

10. If there is a particular day in the week when you will not be able to work in the kitchen, be sure that all the foods in your menu for the day are prepared ahead of time.

11. Make sure you understand all the rules of the diet before you go on it. Read the rules and principles carefully.

12. Learn how to use the "Food Family Chart" (Appendix D) so you can easily make the correct substitutions for any foods you choose not to eat. Plan and purchase the substitute foods in advance so *all* of the food you need will be available.

13. Carry your menu plan for the day with you and make a commitment to yourself—and the soon-to-be new, thinner you—to stay with it. It helps to copy each day's foods and the day's menu plan on a small card and put it in your pocket. Copying this information is good psychology because it sets the food list and the idea of eating only those specific foods in your mind. And you will always have it to refer to if needed.

SHOPPING AND FOOD PREPARATION

14. Clean out your refrigerator, freezer, and pantry shelves by removing all temptations. If they are not there, it is much easier on you.

15. Before you begin the diet, make a list of all of the staple items needed. We always keep an adequate supply of the different whole grains, nuts, seeds, oils, dried fruits, and a few frozen, out-of-season fruits and vegetables on hand.

16. Shop every three days so all of your food will be fresh and delicious-looking in addition to being tasty. Food that looks good is much more satisfying.

17. For variety and convenience, you may want to try different forms of the same food. Look at your list of foods and think about the different forms they are available in. Nuts, for example, can be bought as nut butters, whole, chopped, ground, or pressed for their oils. Grains come in cereal form, whole or ground for cooking, or puffed or flaked to eat cold. They can often be found as a form of cracker, like rice cakes (from brown rice), unflavored rye crackers, or matzohs (wheat and water). Fruits can be eaten whole, dried, stewed, pureed, frozen, or in juice form. Avoid canned fruits and vegetables as much as possible. Vegetables may be eaten raw, lightly steamed (with the cooking water saved), pureed, or juiced. Make sure all prepared foods have nothing added to them.

18. Be adventurous and try all the foods on the diet. One of the main ideas of the diet is to give you an opportunity to eat foods that you have rarely or never eaten before. You will probably find that you like most of them very much. Think of these new tastes and textures as part of your culinary education.

19. Visit your local health-food and specialty stores. They have an interesting variety of foods you have not eaten before. Go in and look around, become familiar with their products, and ask questions. Try foods that look good to you on the days those particular foods appear on the diet.

20. Grow your own seeds and bean sprouts. It is easy to do and fun to watch them sprout; they are delicious and very nutritious. Buy the best starting materials available at your health-food store and discuss sprouting with the manager.

21. Experiment with sugars. Maple sugar and maple syrup are delicious on foods; also available are rice sugar, date sugar, and many types of honey. Shop for these sugars in your health-food store. Don't forget banana chips, currants, raisins, other dried fruits, and the naturally sweet juices as natural sweeteners.

22. Herb teas may be bought in your health-food store. Many supermarkets have them, too. Try a selection of them. They are quite flavorful and have no caffeine. You may drink one with one of your meals each day, but be sure to rotate them and to separate family members properly. And avoid special herb mixtures.

23. If you can tolerate soy, you can buy tofu, soybeans, soy nuts, soy oil, and tamari (wheat-free only) and use them as often as once in four days. Soy is a protein-rich food. The fermented soybean food called "tempeh" is not only a complete protein but also one of the few vegetable foods containing vitamin B_{12}. This will be helpful to vegetarians planning their protein on the diet.

24. Finger foods are perfect to take for lunch. Most fruits and whole or sliced vegetables taste good cold. They can also be steamed, seasoned, and taken along in a glass container to be eaten later. Fresh fruits, of course, can be eaten as they are, and so can nuts, seeds, and dried fruits. Hot foods can be carried in a Thermos.

25. Buy fresh fish from a fish market that you can trust. The gills should be bright, pinkish-red, not brown or blue (don't be squeamish—lift the gill flaps to see); the eyes should be bright, not glazed or pushed in. The bellies should be firm and bounce back into place after being touched. They should smell fresh, not "fishy."

26. Get into the habit of reading labels. There are so many hidden ingredients in packaged foods, and the advertising may be misleading or deceptive. Beware of products marked "all natural" and read their labels carefully before buying them. Ingredients are listed on labels in order of their relative quantities in the package. If water is listed first, then there is more water than anything else, and so on down the list of ingredients. Remember, even if the chemicals are listed last and you say to yourself, "There is so little BHT [or BHA or sodium benzoate or coloring, etc.], how can that hurt me?"—it can and will hurt you if you are sensitive to it.

    A "natural" flavor may be combined with an artificial color. You cannot trust the word "natural" appearing on a label in deceptively large print. Read the small print, too; the culprits are hidden there.

    Reading labels will also teach you the hidden sources of foods that have been causing your problems. Did you know that wheat can be found not only in the obvious foods like bread, cake, and pasta, but in barley malt (beer), licorice and other candies, hamburgers, ice cream, liverwurst, bouillon, soy sauce, vitamin E, mayonnaise, Ovaltine, Postum, soups, and some yeast? Or that sugar can be found in ketchup, beer, mayonnaise, mouthwash, salad dressing, wine, and salt? Appendix F at the back of the book lists some of the common sources of hidden food allergens.

27. Do your diet in style so you don't feel deprived for one minute. Linda Beckwith carries her spring water with her in a Vandermint liqueur bottle and feels elegantly stylish.

    Preparing our recipes will make you feel you are eating special gourmet meals. They are both tempting to look at and delicious to eat, yet simple to prepare. So treat yourself to them regularly.

28. Stay on the diet exactly as it is printed for the first three weeks (unless some foods make you too uncomfortable and must be eliminated). After that time, you may make substitutions or deletions as desired.

29. Keep a food diary. Every time you feel uncomfortable, make a note of the exact symptoms next to the food or foods you just ate. You will find this information indispensable in determining which foods cause your cravings, binges, overeating, fluid retention, and fat storage.

30. Be prepared for temptations and taste-bud seductions. Sandra Boogertman tells us that she is never hungry on the diet except when her hunger is "turned on" by someone offering her candy, pie, or cookies. If you should begin to think about those foods, direct your mind to your goals and the rewards you will have from being thin. Then immediately separate yourself from the source of the temptation, drink a glass of water, and forget about the food.

31. Eat slowly, chew your food thoroughly, and enjoy your meals. When you feel satisfied, stop eating, even if there is some food left on your plate and you know that you could finish it. This can be difficult because you may feel guilty about leaving the food, but it will look better on the plate than on your hips.

32. Don't cook for others when you are hungry. If you are tempted to "taste" what you are cooking, eat before you prepare foods for your family.

33. Exercise every day. You will get some energy from your stored fat and lose weight faster. There is nothing like losing weight fast to keep you on the diet.

34. Drink water when you feel hungry. It can decrease your cravings for food—and if you are a smoker, it will reduce your need for a cigarette.

35. If you "must" have a food that is not on the day's menu, cleverly trick yourself the way arthritis patient Carol Gaudreault does. She knows that it only tastes good for a minute, so instead of eating, she *pretends* to eat it. She imagines that she is eating it, mentally bites it, chews it, tastes it—and then feels as if she has eaten it. "And if I've already eaten it, my need for it is gone."

36. Brushing your teeth after meals is helpful. It makes your mouth feel fresh and puts a sweet end to a meal.

37. If you find yourself in the middle of a food binge, stop eating immediately. Leave the kitchen. Go out for a walk or into the bedroom and take a nap. Go back on the diet immediately.

Make a note in your food diary of the food that set the binge off and avoid it for at least five days. When you do eat it, eat it cautiously and be ready for the cravings.

38. Think of how much better you feel because of being on the diet. Maxine Rolnick says it was no problem to stay on even the Every Meal's a Test Meal Diet, because she felt terrible if she went off it. On it, she was losing weight and feeling well. Marlene Shone keeps from being bored with one food per meal by occasionally eating an allergenic food that causes a reaction. "Then I remember why I should follow my diet."

DEALING WITH SOCIAL PRESSURES

39. Do not permit social pressure to "make" you go off the diet. You must protect your needs and say, "It's for my health and self-image."
40. If you have a family, get them on the diet, too. This will be easy with the It's Not Your Fault You're Fat Diet because the recipes are so good. The Every Meal's a Test Meal Diet is a little more difficult. While you are eating one food at each meal, you could give your family several of the foods listed for that meal. Or, you could use the It's Not Your Fault You're Fat Diet for your family menu. Make a full meal for them and choose a single food for yourself.
41. When you are going to a party, call in advance and say that you are on a diet. Once you have announced that, you wouldn't dare cheat! Bring finger foods of the day with you to snack on. Many of our dieting patients and friends have elaborate social engagements to attend. Estherelka Kaplan, the wife of Canada's solicitor general, Robert Kaplan, often has to give or go to important dinners for the Canadian government. When she gives the dinner, she includes some of the foods from the diet in her menus. When she goes out, she may eat part of her scheduled food at home and then is very careful at the dinner. At times she may move some food around her plate to make it look as if she has eaten more than she actually has.

John Barritt, Speaker of the House of Bermuda, says there are some occasions when he must take a drink, but he drinks only water, even if he is making a toast. Mr. Barritt says, "You've got to make a commitment. Say to yourself, 'I am going to do this.' It's worth sticking to the course. There's not much point starting unless you're going to finish."

DEALING WITH CIGARETTE SMOKE

42. Try an invisible nasal filter, available at pharmacies.
43. If there is a lot of smoke, stand near the doorway, window, or a fan, and step out of the room frequently.
44. Don't allow any smoking in your home, office, or car. Make it clear that you are allergic to smoke. People really don't mind stepping outside to smoke. Post a "Thank You For Not Smoking" sign and do not provide any ashtrays.

EATING AT RESTAURANTS

45. Choose a restaurant likely to have the foods that are on your diet for that day. Some days on the It's Not Your Fault You're Fat Diet are keyed to ethnic foods—Chinese, Japanese, Greek, Italian, or French. Check your menu for the day and then choose the restaurant.
46. Order your foods cooked plain—with no butter, sauce, or gravy—and inform the waiter that this is absolutely necessary or you will not be able to eat the food.
47. Don't forget that coffee and tea are nonnutritive, drug-containing "foods" that must be rotated. You may carry herb-tea bags with you and order a pot of hot water if you like a hot drink after meals.
48. Remember that you can drink club soda, seltzer, or mineral water. And don't overlook single-food fruit or vegetable juices in rotation.

COLLEGE DORMS

49. You can keep in your room finger-food snacks on the diet that do not need refrigeration. Explain your diet to the dorm dietitian and ask if you can have your protein food cooked without sauces or other ingredients. You may have trouble trying to stay on the It's Not Your Fault You're Fat Diet, but you could easily follow the Every Meal's a Test Meal Diet.

MAINTENANCE

After losing all the weight you want to, the challenge is to keep it off. Our maintenance diet is one you can live on. It is a healthy diet for you and your family; and with just a little discipline, you can stay within its limits. A few tips:

50. Weigh yourself faithfully every morning. If you have gained more than 2 pounds, you know you have done too much cheating. You now know why you gain weight and how to painlessly keep it from happening. If you allow yourself to eat foods that lead you to eat compulsively, there is no one else to blame but you, and it *will be* your fault you're fat!

51. As soon as you detect the very first hint of food cravings of addictive eating, get back on Day 1 of your diet immediately.

52. Keep your worst offenders completely out of your life for at least two or three months. If you do regain tolerance of them, be careful to eat them only once a week. You will feel so much better physically and mentally when you avoid those foods you are allergic to.

53. Most of all, at all times remain aware of your improved appearance, increased sense of well-being, and the relationship of these important benefits to your diet. Remember what can happen if you don't take care of yourself. Decide to be your own best friend and keep yourself healthy and slim.

12

QUESTIONS AND ANSWERS

IS THIS DIET FOR ME?

How many people have food allergies?

Based on the experience of 300 clinical ecologists (the food-allergy and environmental experts), the estimates range from a low of 50% up to 90%. Clinical ecologists use more accurate methods of testing for food allergies and food addictions than traditional allergists, and we are able to diagnose many cases that the conventional allergists fail to identify. We have clinical proof that food allergy is a major medical problem that is an important part of many physical and mental disorders.

Are there some foods that almost everyone is allergic to?

There are no foods that everyone is allergic to, but there are a number of foods that allergic people often react to. These are the foods we eat frequently. Milk is the leading offender in children; coffee in adults. After those come wheat, eggs, apples, bananas, beef, beet sugar, black pepper, cane sugar, chicken, chocolate, corn, lettuce, mustard, oats, onions, oranges, peanuts, pork, potatoes, rice, rye, soy, string beans, tea, tomatoes, and tuna.

How likely is it that food allergy is the source of my overweight?

It is very likely. Overweight is usually the result of overeating combined with fluid retention. Allergic food addiction causes you to crave food and eat more calories than you need. Excess calories are stored in the body as fat deposits.

Fluid retention is another common allergic condition. During an allergic reaction, the thin-walled capillaries (small blood vessels) throughout your body will leak fluid into the surrounding tissues and cause edema, which shows up as excess body weight. Unless you can rid yourself of the edema, it is difficult to lose weight. This is why so many undiagnosed or misdiagnosed cases of food allergy are taking "water pills" daily.

Are there other biological reasons why it may be difficult for me to lose weight?

Yes. There are some overweight people whose metabolism is not functioning normally. Their doctors may have told them that they have a hypothyroid problem. It is the thyroid's function to regulate the body's rate of metabolism. If a person's thyroid gland is underactive, he or she is not "burning" calories at a normal rate. Overweight could certainly be a result of this condition.

How many people have been on this diet?

The Rotary Diversified Diet was devised by Dr. Herbert Rinkel almost fifty years ago. Since then, allergists (who later became clinical ecologists) have had remarkable success with tens of thousands of patients.

Both diets in this book and the maintenance diet are based on principles of the Rotary Diversified Diet. Every overweight person who has tested them has lost weight more easily than they ever believed possible.

I'm on the go all day long; I travel in my work. The menu plans and recipes of the It's Not Your Fault You're Fat Diet seem so elaborate—and I don't think I could manage on one food per meal. Is this diet for me?

Our diet is portable, and the recipes are simple to prepare. Most of them can be cooked ahead of time and eaten hot or cold. Many of the raw and dried foods—like vegetables, fruits, seeds, nuts, and sprouts—can be carried with you. The key to the diet is planning and preparation. Know what you have to eat each day and always keep it available, or know where to go eat.

I'm a vegetarian. Both diets list many meats, shellfish, fish, and fowl. Can I go on this diet without eating them?

Yes. Since the It's Not Your Fault You're Fat Diet does not require that you eat all of the foods listed for the day, simply eliminate the meats, fish, and fowl, and increase the quantities of grains, beans, seeds, and nuts.

We would prefer that vegetarians not go on the Every Meal's a Test Meal Diet unless you are willing to eat fish or shellfish. That diet does not allow you to combine vegetables to make the whole proteins that your body needs for continuous muscle and organ repair, maintenance, and growth as you lose weight.

Fish appears often on this diet, and I don't like fish. Any ideas?

The reason many adults do not like fish is that they have unpleasant childhood memories of odorous and "fishy-tasting" seafood. If you are past 40, the fish you ate as a child was probably poorly refrigerated. Also, some fish have a naturally strong taste. We suggest you give fish a fair trial by eating freshly caught, mild-tasting species such as sole, flounder, scrod, haddock, and swordfish, and be sure not to overcook it (see Appendix B). You will be surprised by the mild, delicate flavor of a properly cooked, freshly caught fish.

Can I afford the It's Not Your Fault You're Fat Diet?

If you buy all the foods on the diet and shop carefully, the diet should cost you about $7 a day. If that is too expensive, you can substitute less-expensive foods for the higher-priced foods. We have given you a choice of fish when more expensive seafood appears. Remember, this diet is an adventure in healthy eating and will have many long-term health benefits. Expensive foods like chestnuts, maple sugar, some of the dried fruit, and fresh fruits and vegetables out of season can be either omitted for the day, substituted for, or bought frozen. We know that if you want to go on the diet, you will find the right way for you.

I have stopped smoking many times, and I gained weight and went back to smoking each time. How can you demand that in order to lose weight I have to stop smoking "cold turkey"?

This is the best time to quit smoking. Many of our patients find it is not too difficult once they have made up their minds—if they take enough springwater and vitamin C, which help clear nicotine and chemical residues out of the system, reducing tobacco cravings. Rotating foods breaks your food cravings (which may cause the restless irritability that you smoke to relieve). The sugar added to tobacco and the chemicals in tobacco smoke are potent causes of your food cravings. In short, your cigarettes can be an important contributing factor to your weight problems; they are chemical offenders.

I find a daily drink relaxes me after a hard day. Must I give it up?

If you really must have a drink in order to be comfortable, you probably are addicted to some ingredient in your "daily drink." That end-of-day tension you feel is probably due to withdrawal symptoms, not stresses at work. In order to test your reactions to foods—including those from which your favorite alcoholic beverage is made—you must give up alcohol for at least the first two weeks of this diet. After that, you may test your reactions to wine, sake, rum, or pure Russian vodka on days when grapes, rice, cane sugar, or potatoes, respectively, are allowed.

Other drinks—such as scotch, rye, gin, bourbon, and beer—have many ingredients in them. It is best not to test them until you have tested most of the foods on the diet and found that you tolerate yeast and at least all of the grains as well. By that time, you may find that you no longer have a need for alcohol.

Is this diet safe for pregnant women?

A pregnant woman should consult her doctor before she embarks on any diet. She needs a diet rich in nutrients to maintain her health and that of her baby. Pregnancy is *not* the time for a woman to be concerned about her weight. Recent findings indicate that a pregnant woman should eat and drink in response to her physiologic needs, and a weight gain of 25 to 40 pounds is regarded as normal.

However, a pregnant woman with multiple food allergies can do herself and her unborn baby a great service by eating foods in rotation (but only after consulting her doctor). This will minimize or eliminate the effects of food allergy. She may use the It's Not Your Fault You're Fat Diet for that purpose—except that she should eat whatever quantities of foods will satisfy her hunger and not worry about the scale. She must avoid harmful chemical exposures, especially tobacco smoke. And alcoholic beverages are prohibited, since it has been established that alcohol may have an extremely serious effect on the unborn child's developing nervous system.

Is the It's Not Your Fault You're Fat Diet safe for young children?

This is the healthiest diet you and anyone in your family can be on. Young children and other family members will enjoy the diet with no restrictions on how much they can eat of each food. You, of course, have to lose weight and want to keep your food intake within the confines of the diet.

A food-rotation habit is one of the most valuable health measures that you can teach a family member. And, it will last a lifetime.

I have been diagnosed as having reactive hypoglycemia. I notice that your diets include many high-carbohydrate foods. Are these diets really safe for me?

Yes, our diets are safe for you.

Although you have been diagnosed as having hypoglycemia, this is rarely the correct diagnosis. Marshall has seen hundreds of such patients at the Center, and he has conclusively shown that, in most instances, reactive hypoglycemia is a misdiagnosed case of addictive food allergy. In addition, he has frequently caused so-called hypoglycemic symptoms during testing with high-protein foods.

You cannot know whether or not you will have any symptoms after you consume any of the high-carbohydrate foods until you have tested your personal, biologically unique response to each individual high-carbohydrate food. Apples, bananas, dates, figs, apricots, pears, potatoes, yams, millet, rice, wheat, etc., must be eaten in proper rotation in a sequence of single-food test meals in order to clearly demonstrate their effects, if any, on each person.

If you are concerned about the possibility of a severe or uncomfortable reaction from certain foods, do your first single-food ingestion tests with small portions of each of the "suspect" foods. If a one-quarter serving of a regular portion of a food is well tolerated, you should take progressively larger portions of that food each time it comes up in the diet. If your rotational series of eating tests shows that you react to one or several specific high-carbohydrate foods—or any other kind—you must temporarily eliminate these offenders from your diet as soon as they are identified. You will probably find there are many well-tolerated "safe" carbohydrate foods that you have unnecessarily eliminated because you believed that you were hypoglycemic!

I have been on a special diet in which I eat a limited number of foods very often. Can eating this way have any harmful effects?

Any diet in which a limited number of foods are eaten daily or several times a day—such as the multiple feedings of high-protein foods in "hypoglycemia"—constitutes an overexposure to those particular foods. It is quite possible that this dietary overloading has caused you to become allergically addicted to some or many of those foods. This explains why you, and many other "hypoglycemics," do not feel well when you do not eat your addicting foods early enough to block or mask withdrawal symptoms that appear when you are late for a meal. This also explains how those favorite foods appear to give you energy, increased alertness, or a sense of well-being. The rotary diversified diets in this book will help you to unmask your food addictions and lose the weight they have been causing. Consult your doctor before changing any prescribed dietary regimen you may be following at present.

I'm very overweight, and the only way I've been able to lose weight in the past is to fast—but I gain the weight right back. Will I really be able to lose weight eating ten foods a day?

Yes. The reason you gain your weight back is because as soon as you begin to eat, you go back to eating your old favorites, which are probably the foods you are allergically addicted to. These foods cause you to eat compulsively and retain water at the same time. For the majority of overweight individuals, these are the most important factors in gaining weight.

Our diets, in conjunction with environmental changes and appropriate allergy management, eliminate compulsive eating and water-retention problems. You will lose weight and keep it off as long as you follow the instructions in the book.

Will the medications I am presently taking interfere with losing weight on this diet?

Do not discontinue any medications that your personal physician has prescribed unless he or she authorizes you to do so. But please try to eliminate over-the-counter drugs that you have elected to take without your doctor's knowledge—especially appetite-control drugs or "water pills" that you may be taking to lose weight. When this diet helps you to lose weight and feel better, tell your physician about it. If your doctor has an open mind, he or she will be pleased to learn how foods affect you, especially if you can turn "puzzling" symptoms on and off as you also lose weight. It is vital information that you should share with him or her because it will enable your doctor to help others with similar problems.

Is there anyone who should not go on this diet?

Yes. Because a Rotary Diversified Diet can produce flare-ups of any familiar symptoms. If you have had any condition which could be life-threatening, you must not go on this diet without clearing it with a qualified physician. Life-threatening conditions include suicidal depression or violent, uncontrollable rages, as well as severe asthma requiring emergency treatment, diabetes, or severe epileptic seizures.

However, if you are in generally good health, with only mild to moderate day-to-day aches, pains, or mood swings, there is little chance you will get into difficulty.

I have been in the habit of fasting occasionally for the sake of my health. May I continue to do so while on the It's Not Your Fault You're Fat Diet?

Certainly. Omitting an occasional meal, or going on a one-day fast when you can do so comfortably, is a highly effective way to burn off some stored fat, and you may do so as long as your doctor approves. Our diet will eliminate your compulsive eating patterns, and on days when your decreased appetite is not reminding you to eat, a short fast will help bring you to your objective ahead of schedule. If you are in good condition, and your doctor approves, a longer fast, if you are so inclined, is another way to break addictive eating patterns, lose retained fluids, use up extra calories from your fat deposits, and bring about the diagnostically valuable state of increased sensitivity that is necessary for accurate single-food testing.

FOLLOWING THE DIRECTIONS

What preparation is needed before I go on this diet?

First, consult with your doctor. Read the rules carefully and look over the diet plan.

Second, make a shopping list. List all of the staple items needed for the first week, such as grains, oils, dried fruits, nuts, and seeds, Add to that list the fresh meats, fish, fruits, and vegetables for the first three days. If you are going to the health-food store, you might call them to find out the prices of the foods you intend to buy so you can plan a budget.

Third, make up your mind that you will have the discipline to follow the rules for weight loss and greater health. It is easy. Good luck.

I don't like to cook. Do I have to prepare all of the foods you suggest in the It's Not Your Fault You're Fat Diet?

You may eat only the foods we suggest, but it is not necessary that you eat all of them. You may not eat foods that are not listed. The diets have been very carefully planned for you. If you want to eliminate some foods for the day, do not eliminate the high-protein foods. A large part of your body structure is composed of protein and you require an intake of between 8 and 12 ounces a day of high-quality protein foods like meat, fish, and poultry to maintain your protein balance. If you do not eat enough protein, you will use some of your own muscle tissue to meet your needs. You are not required to use our recipes. They are there for your convenience. We suggest that you try them. They are simple and make your eating experiences much more enjoyable.

May I use two forms of the same food in the same meal?

Yes. If you want to use the different textures of the same foods, you may crunch into an apple, eat applesauce, and drink apple juice in the same meal; or eat peanuts, unsweetened peanut butter, and use peanut oil. The choice is yours as long as the different forms of the food remain in the same meal. Many of the menu plans utilize foods in this way.

May I drink an herbal tea throughout the day as a substitute for water?

No. Spring water is the only beverage you may take any time you wish. Herbs are biologically distinct foods; and like all other foods, each must be taken only once in each rotation cycle—at one meal— with a minimum interval of four days before it is repeated in your diet. It must be taken on alternate days from other foods in the same family. Choose which meal you want to enjoy with a cup of herb tea. Of course, you may have more than one cup at that time. Do not drink a mixture of blended herbs, however, because if you take too many herbs at once, there may not be enough remaining herbs to permit a different tea selection several times in a rotation cycle. This also applies to herbs and spices that are used with other foods.

I have a terrible "sweet tooth." I don't like to drink herb teas (not to mention coffee or tea) without sugar. What do you suggest?

Your sweet tooth will not go unfed on this diet. Each day has sweets in the form of dried fruits or maple syrup or honey. If your "sweet of the day" comes in sugar form (like date sugar, maple sugar, or rice sugar), you may choose to use that in your tea; otherwise, you will have to enjoy your tea without adding sugar to it. (Try eating a dried fruit with it for sweetness.) You may have only the herb tea listed for the day. Coffee and tea are nonnutritious, drug-containing beverages that do you no good and are best avoided. They are permitted, but not recommended, once every four to seven days.

I have some favorite herbs and spices not used in the recipes. May I substitute them?

For the first three weeks, it's best to follow our diets exactly as they are written. Then, after you know which foods and meals you have no reaction to, you certainly may substitute other foods, including herbs or spices. Follow the rules for substitution in chapter 9. Herbs and spices can cause a lot of mischief if they are not carefully rotated with related foods as well as other herbs or spices.

I'm on a low-salt diet for my blood pressure. May I still use sea salt?

Do what your doctor tells you in this matter, and ask your doctor about salt substitutes. (You may find that certain spices or herbs will give you the extra flavor you're looking for.) Keep in mind that many people who lose weight will also have a significant drop in their blood pressure without even reducing their sodium intake. It is a good idea to have your blood pressure checked during our diets because you may be pleasantly surprised to learn that it is lower. This can be due to both weight loss and elimination of food allergies that cause increased blood pressure.[1]

I know I will feel terrible about not eating my leftovers the next day. Do I have to stick strictly to the diet?

Yes. Don't worry about the leftovers. Freeze them or feed them to a

---

[1] For a discussion of the allergic factor in high blood pressure, see *Dr. Mandell's 5-Day Allergy Relief System* (New York: Pocket Books, 1980).

family member. You are doing this for your health, which is more important. You will soon learn to prepare just the right amount of food.

What if I want to eat a food not listed in the menu plans for either diet?

Follow the diet as listed for at least twenty-one days, if at all possible. Then, substitute any food or foods you wish according to the rules for substitution in the chapter on the diet. Use the "Eat Anywhere" foods (Appendix E) and refer to the "Food Family Chart" (Appendix D) for additional ideas.

How important is it to keep a food diary? It seems like a bother to carry it around, and I'm sure I'll remember bad reactions.

Your food diary is a very important diagnostic tool. It is a permanent record of your reactions and it identifies your particular definite, probable, and suspected food offenders. The only way you can be sure you'll remember your reactions to each food is to write them down as they occur. We can guarantee that with the passage of time, and one food reaction following another, the time will come when your memory will fail you and those overlapping "I'll never forget this one" reactions will blend into each other.

There are other things to note in your food diary, too. Note where you were when you developed symptoms, because exposures to environmental factors can cause the same reactions that foods do. After all, they eventually get into your system after you breathe them into the body. Note whether your reaction was mild, moderate, or severe. This will help you plan the foods to eat and avoid on the diet.

What do I do if I react after a meal?

If you feel moderately uncomfortable, you may obtain relief from a food reaction by using any of the home remedies in chapter 7. The remedies include vitamin C, Alka-Seltzer "Gold," sodium bicarbonate, a short nap, a laxative, or an enema if necessary.

If I'm still reacting to one food, do I have to wait until the reaction is over before eating again?

Yes, to avoid the confusion of trying to distinguish between a prolonged reaction and two overlapping reactions, you must wait for a reaction to subside before eating again. If you are still reacting to one food when you eat another, you cannot be certain which food is causing which symptoms, and you will have to repeat the tests at greater intervals in the future.

For future reference, record your reactions in your food diary.

What if I react twice in a row to the same food—but with a different reaction?

It is not unusual for a food-allergic person's reaction to a food to vary. On one day, that food might make your throat itch; on another, your throat might be sore and you might also have a stuffy nose—or you might get a headache instead of the sore throat because you were more or less tired and were exposed to some other factors that you also react to.

Did you buy a different brand or form of the food, and did this one have some chemicals in it? Did you eat it at a restaurant this time, whereas previously you had cooked it at home? Perhaps you are reacting because of a heavy exposure to tobacco smoke in the restaurant—or to a seasoning the restaurant added despite your request for the "pure" food. Retest the food one or more times when it comes up again in the diet and you may be able to clarify this situation. Look back through your food diary for clues. But don't worry about it if the symptoms were only mild ones.

If I find I react to one food in a family, does that mean I can't eat the other foods you refer to as being "allergically identical" to it? What about other foods in the same family?

Every allergic person is a one-of-a-kind, biologically unique individual, and his or her reactions to anything are not 100% predictable. The only way to obtain accurate information about your possible reaction to any food is to test it as a single-food feeding challenge.

Chances are greater that people will react to an "allergically identical" food, but this may not be so for you. Some people who are allergic to wheat, for example, can eat very closely related grains in the same botanic tribe such as barley or rye or millet or triticale, and some cannot. You must test each food individually for yourself. If zucchini squash in the gourd family bothers you, cantaloupe and watermelon—closely related but not "identical"—may be perfectly all right. Do not automatically eliminate any of them—try them and be sure.

When I know I'm allergic to a food on the It's Not Your Fault You're Fat Diet, how do I figure out what food to substitute for it?

You may substitute for any food on the diet according to the rules for substitution on pages 157–158. To summarize those rules: "Eat Anywhere" foods may be added on any day, at any time, as long as you do not eat them more than once in four days. All other foods may be substituted on a particular day, as long as you eliminate them from all meals on the three days before and the three days after the day on which you want to eat them. In addition, you must be sure not to eat foods in the same family any closer together than on alternate days. Rotate them on a two-day basis. Refer to the "Food Family Chart," Appendix D.

If I lose weight and my blood pressure goes down, must I continue blood-pressure medication?

Weight loss is frequently associated with lowered blood pressure. Many physicians have indicated that losing weight may be the only treatment needed to lower blood pressure into the normal range.

Once your blood pressure is normal and hypertension ceases to exist, antihypertension medications may no longer be indicated. It is possible, however, that your physician may feel otherwise, and since he or she is thoroughly familiar with your condition, it is in your best interest to consult with him or her about this matter. It would be appropriate for you to discuss reducing the dosage of your medication if your pressure has had a modest improvement during early phases of this diet.

I've heard that allergies can be overcome by good nutrition. Do you recommend any particular food supplements?

It is true that good nutrition and nutritional supplements (vitamins and minerals) can help many people to reduce the number and severity of their allergies. That is one of the reasons why this diet emphasizes good, wholesome, fresh foods like whole grains, fresh fruits and vegetables, organically grown produce, and cold-pressed oils—and why we eliminate refined flour and refined sugar (except to test them), white rice, and the additives found in processed and packaged foods. It's best not to take any food supplements other than pure vitamin C for the first three weeks, so you can see what foods you are sensitive to. After that, consult with your doctor to find a multivitamin and mineral supplement that is free of your particular allergen(s). (See p. 77 for suggestions regarding supplements.)

What if I go off the diet once in a while?

Don't feel guilty—you're only human. It's not the end of the world. But *don't* rationalize that since you've broken the diet, you might as well continue to do so! This is self-destructive—why would you want to lose all the benefits you have already achieved? Just pay Mother Nature whatever price she demands—whatever symptoms you must now suffer, if any—and go right back on the diet. Your body will soon forgive you.

PROBLEMS

How can I find a reliable source of organically grown foods?

Find an organic-food co-op and become a member of it. See if there is a local organic-gardening club and find out if the members have extra produce—or start your own garden. Investigate your local health food stores.

If you cannot get organic food, look for the best-quality fresh, whole, unrefined, unprocessed food you can find, as close to its natural state as possible. Fresh-frozen food is preferable to canned. Stay away from preservatives, chemicals, additives, artificial flavorings and colorings. Avoid packaged food mixtures. Cook your food from scratch.

I've just started the diet and I'm sticking to it—but I find I'm eating large amounts of food. Can I really lose weight this way?

Don't worry about eating too much in the first week or so of the diet. As your food addictions disappear, so will the compulsive eating that has kept you overweight. Just stay on the diet exactly as it is written, especially the first three weeks. You will find your hunger will decrease significantly during the first three to five days. Soon, you will be surprised at how little food you will need and want to eat.

Why is it that I can eat some foods raw and not have reactions, but if I eat them cooked, I react? Conversely, there are some foods I can eat cooked with no reaction, but I react when I eat them raw.

This is not an uncommon situation among food-allergic individuals. Heating definitely changes the allergic properties of some foods.

The rules say not to eat more often than once in four hours, and to eat just enough to satisfy one's appetite—not to overeat. But knowing that I won't be eating again for four hours, I sometimes eat more than I need to feel satisfied. Can I shorten the time between meals?

No. Hunger in itself does not cause an important degree of discomfort. You think that it is hunger that you fear, but it is probably the symptoms you associate with hunger—the withdrawal symptoms of food addiction, such as headaches, grogginess, irritability, or tension—that you are concerned about. You should *not* eat to alleviate those symptoms; instead, take Alka-Seltzer "Gold" as directed, and if there is no relief, take vitamin C in spring water (which should hold you until it's time for the next meal). If you can, lie down to rest for a little while until the symptoms clear up.

I'm in the first week of the diet and I feel terrible. What's going on? Are you sure this diet is healthy?

Yes, it is healthy. This diet cannot flare up any health problems that you do not already have, but you may never have realized that you had important food-related symptoms. You are experiencing a heightened form of your unrecognized addictive food allergies. Stick it out—these withdrawal pangs will not last, and you will feel much better soon, and will find out which foods are causing your discomfort as you test them one at a time in rotation.

On some days, I feel very uncomfortable. I thought you said I'd feel better after the first five days of withdrawal symptoms. What's going on?

Those "bad" days after the withdrawal period are probably caused by acute reactions to foods that you have not eaten for at least four days. Remember, because you have avoided them, you are now hypersensitive to foods you were addicted to, and these now-unmasked offenders are easy to flare up.

Remember, *this diet cannot cause any new symptoms.* Your reactions are the acute form of the allergic addiction you were suppressing (masking) by regularly eating the food(s) that you are now reacting to. When you identify which foods you are allergic to, take them out of your diet for a couple of months. **BUT IF YOU BEGIN TO HAVE MEDICAL PROBLEMS ABOVE AND BEYOND THOSE WE'VE DISCUSSED, CONSULT YOUR DOCTOR.**

What if I find that I react to every food I test?

You may be what we call a "universal food reactor"—one of those not so rare people who react to a very wide variety of foods—just about every food that you eat. It is also possible that you are reacting to the chemicals involved in the production and processing of foods. In this case, organically grown foods may be helpful. On a self-help program, it will be necessary for you to eat those foods that caused the mildest symptoms; and if you find there are not enough foods of known safety, you must eat those that cause mild to moderate reactions.

If you cannot construct an adequate diet from the foods that give you mild to moderate reactions, it is possible you may be able to tolerate game meats. Many are available at special stores or by mail-order catalog, such as Czimmer Food, Inc., Rural Route 1, Box 285, Lockport, Illinois 60441, phone (815) 838-3503. They will be happy to send you their current catalog and price list. A friend or neighbor who hunts may be able to supply you with some game from hunting trips; the local Rifle Association may also be able to put you in touch with hunters.

If you find your broad-based food allergy problem is too difficult to solve alone, this is the time to consult with a clinical ecologist. Contact us at the Alan Mandell Center for Bioecologic Diseases, or write to Dr. Del Stigler, Secretary of the Society for Clinical Ecology, at 2005 Franklin, Suite 490, Denver, Colorado 80205, for names of qualified clinical ecologists in your area. Send a self-addressed stamped envelope.

I have been faithfully staying on the diet, but I find I am still overeating compulsively sometimes. This reaction does not seem to be associated with particular foods. What could be the reason?

If you are observing our diet to the letter, there will be no hidden foods to provoke either addictive-compulsive eating or overstimulation of your appetite; therefore, some other factor or factors are responsible. It may be a chemical exposure or it may be an internal response to one of the common airborne allergens, such as mildew in your basement, molds growing in the soil of your potted plants or on a piece of mildewed furniture.

Don't overlook the possibility that there may be chemicals, dust, and molds in your attic, garage, workshop, or hobby room. Some chemicals that can induce and perpetuate addictive eating include cigarette smoke, cosmetics, plastics, housekeeping and laundry supplies, heating fuels and their combustion products, and numerous chemical air pollutants that are encountered outdoors and at work.

There are one or two foods that I just can't resist. What if I keep eating them?

If you do not rid yourself of a current addiction, the problem will undoubtedly get worse with the passage of time. Use a little discipline to get to the root of your problem and eliminate it.

I was losing weight steadily for two months, but now my weight has been the same for several weeks. What should I do?

For reasons not fully understood, some people run into temporary plateaus where there is no further weight loss for a short time—and then the progressive weight loss begins again as they continue on the diet. Other individuals will have made internal adjustments in their utilization of food (metabolism), which make them much more efficient "food processors." For those individuals, increased exercise and/or a lower caloric intake is necessary to achieve further weight reduction by burning excess body fat for energy.

I've been on the Every Meal's a Test Meal Quick Weight Loss Diet for two weeks. I've learned a lot about my reactions to foods, but my digestive system is acting up a lot. Is this an allergic reaction? I don't usually have such problems.

You may be having allergic reactions to many of the foods you are eating. The diet may have unmasked digestive-tract allergies that you were unaware of because they were covered up all the time by your former eating habits. Or you may find, as a few of our patients have, that your digestive system just functions better when you eat more than one food at a time.

My allergist says I couldn't be allergic to all the foods I find I'm having reactions to. Why do you and he differ?

The skin tests used by traditional allergists for the detection of food allergy are not all reliable, and I (Marshall) do not use them. I discontinued conventional skin testing in my practice about twenty years ago because much more accurate methods of diagnosis were available. There is an 80% diagnostic error when the skin-test technique or the considerably more expensive RAST tests are employed to diagnose food allergy. These tests are performed to demonstrate the presence of antibodies that combine with the foods and cause symptoms. However, the vast majority of food-allergic individuals do not have demonstrable antibodies to the foods that make them ill. Foods responsible for important disorders throughout the body do not always give rise to the production of antibodies that the skin and RAST tests are designed to detect.

Provocative testing with food extracts is 80% *accurate* in demonstrating food-related disorders, because these tests actually reproduce the patients' familiar symptoms. (Allergy extracts for testing do not contain all the factors present in a food, and for that reason some food allergens may be missed—accounting for the other 20%.) **If a food can make you ill, the presence or absence of antibodies to that food is of no practical value to you in terms of managing your illness.** In thousands of instances, I have confirmed these test results by deliberate feeding tests that conclusively prove the relationship between the ingestion of a food and the symptoms it causes. These feeding challenges have been done at home and in the hospital in over 100,000 patients by fellow ecologists.

Finally, many cases of food allergy are of the hidden (masked) variety that smolder along as chronic symptoms, without acute flare-ups, after an offending food has been eaten. *Unfortunately, most traditional, mainstream allergists are not aware of this extremely important and very common form of food allergy. Therefore, they do not suspect it, look for it, or diagnose it even though they encounter such disorders every day.*

FOLLOW-UP

May I stay on the It's Not Your Fault You're Fat Diet for as long as I want?

If you are doing well and you like what is happening—your weight loss, better physical and mental-emotional health, control of your increased sense of well-being—there is no reason not to stay on the It's Not Your Fault You're Fat Diet for six, nine, twelve weeks, or much longer, until you reach your goal and are able to maintain your weight loss. The diet has been designed around balanced, nutritious meals of fresh, whole, unprocessed, unrefined foods that provide your basic nutritional requirements.

Is the Every Meal's a Test Meal Diet healthy to stay on for extended periods of time?

The one-food-a-meal phase of the Every Meal's a Test Meal Diet is not meant to be continued indefinitely by people who can tolerate many other foods. If you want to keep testing one food per meal for another three, six, or even nine weeks to enlarge your diet, that's all right, but the single-food-per-meal part of the diet is designed for immediate appetite and weight control as well as for diagnostic purposes, not to serve as a lifetime eating plan for most of our readers.

Only if you are moderately or severely allergic to so many foods that you do not have enough foods to rotate through two- or three-food meals in a four- to seven-day rotation cycle should you continue on the Every Meal's a Test Meal Diet for two to six months. Many clinical ecologists have patients on this diet for years, and this is satisfactory as long as they are eating enough protein and taking their vitamin supplements. You should not stay on this diet for long periods of time, however, unless you are under your doctor's supervision.

What sort of environmental factors should I look for if I suspect that my reactions are to substances in the environment rather than to foods?

Think about the environment you were in when you had your reaction. Were you driving? Were you in a particular shop or a particular neighborhood? Were there pets in the house? Was it unusually dusty? Were you using some new cleaning product or cosmetic? Was there some chemical in your work area? Was the air-conditioner functioning properly? Could there be mold growing in the basement or under the sink? When you identify the suspected cause of your problem, avoid having it as a part of your life (when possible).

I've been on the It's Not Your Fault You're Fat Diet for twelve weeks, and I've lost 30 pounds. Now I want to make sure I maintain my weight. I'm a little afraid that after the discipline of the strict rotation diet, if I go off on my own, I'll gain the weight again. Yet I want to feel freer to eat out, to eat at friends' houses, and so on. What do you suggest?

On the maintenance diet, be just as strict with yourself at home as you have been these twelve weeks. Have fun when you go out with friends, but don't overdo it—and for day-to-day meals out, carry allowed finger foods with you or order allowed simple fare.

Do not fall back into the addictive-compulsive-eating trap. You look and feel too good to blow it! Be sure you strictly rotate the major offenders you identified in the early phase of your diet. Without compulsive eating, your caloric intake will be easily controlled. If you have a flare-up of your fluid-retention problem (or any other symptom), identify and eliminate the cause or go back to a strict food rotation until the excess fluid is eliminated.

If you are sensitive to the pollens of trees, grasses, or weeds, be extra careful with your diet during those periods of increased allergic exposure (hay-fever seasons) when these pollens are present in the air.

I want to clean up my home environment so that there are no chemicals or other allergens in my house that might be bothering me. How do I go about it?

This is an important subject that deserves your very careful attention, and the reader is referred to the list of suggested readings at the end of the book.

All food offenders that have been shown to cause moderate or severe reactions must be eliminated or controlled to minimize your total load of allergic stress. Your exposure to all forms of chemical agents and airborne allergens—dust, mold, animal danders—must be reduced. It is possible that you may need allergy treatments consisting of periodic injections ("allergy shots" or immunotherapy) of allergenic extracts prepared from dust, pollens, molds, animal danders, etc., to control your reaction to airborne allergens.

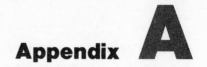

GUIDELINES FOR COOKING GRAINS

In general, grains should be cooked by bringing to a boil 2½ cups of water for every cup of raw grain. Rinse the grain, then stir it into the boiling water with a pinch of salt; make sure that the water is again boiling, cover the pot tightly, and turn heat to low. Cook at low heat, covered, for thirty minutes or until all of the water is absorbed.

Exceptions:
Wild rice takes 1½ cups of water to each cup of grain.
Buckwheat takes only ten minutes to cook.
Millet needs 3 cups of water to every cup of raw grain.

Appendix B

GUIDELINES FOR COOKING FISH

No matter how you decide to cook your fish—whether poaching, broiling, baking, or frying—the same rule applies for judging cooking time:

Measure the width of the fish at the thickest part. Cook it exactly ten minutes at high heat for every inch of width. (If it's three-quarters of an inch thick, cook it exactly seven and a half minutes.)

High heat for broiling means that the fish should be placed two to four inches from the flame or heating element. For baking, it means a temperature of 425° to 450° in the oven. If poaching, start to count the ten minutes from the time when the water starts boiling again after adding the fish.

To measure accurately, lay the fish on its side on a flat surface and place a ruler vertically next to it, the end of the ruler resting on the surface. If you are stuffing the fish, measure its width after stuffing, and if you roll up a fillet, measure the diameter after it is rolled.

Cook frozen fish without first thawing it, but double the cooking time to twenty minutes per inch of thickness.[1]

---

[1]James Beard's *New Fish Cookery* (Boston: Little, Brown, 1976) explains this cooking method in detail. It was developed by the Department of Fisheries of Canada. Beard's cookbook is also an excellent source of ideas for preparing all kinds of seafood.

FOOD DIARY SAMPLE PAGE

Date	Time Food Was Eaten	Food Eaten	Location or Activity at Time of Reaction (Suspected Environmental Factor)	Time of Reaction	Type of Reaction and Its Severity (Mild, Moderate, or Severe)

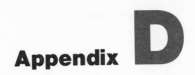

FOOD FAMILY CHART

(Different families are separated by solid horizontal lines. "Allergically identical" foods are enclosed in brackets.)

FISH AND ANIMALS: BIOLOGICALLY RELATED GROUPS

Sea scallop[1]
Bay scallop

Oysters
  Atlantic
  Olympia

Cockle

Clams
  Butter
  Geoduck
  Pismo
  Quahog
  Soft-shell
Mussels

Abalone
  Green
  Pink
  Red

Snail

North American squid

Octopus

Shrimp
  Brown-grooved
  Pink-grooved
Prawn

Lobster
  American
  European
Crayfish

Crab
  European edible
  Dungeness
  Blue

Honeybee (Honey)[2]

Shark

Beluga
Common sturgeon
North American lake
  sturgeon

Oregon/Sacramento
  sturgeon
Caviar

North American paddlefish

Tarpon

Herring
  Atlantic
  Pacific
  Sardine[3]
Manhaden
Shad

Anchovy

Salmon (caviar)
  Atlantic
  Caho
  Dog
  King
  Pink
  Sockeye

---

[1] Imitation sea scallops may be cut from shark or ray with a cookie-cutter-like utensil. Imitation scallops may be served in some restaurants.

[2] Honey contains some bee substance and comes from various flowers.

[3] Sardines are small or half-grown herrings.

Trout
  Brook
  Brown
  Lake
  Rainbow

Lake whitefish

Common smelt

Muskellunge
Northern pike
Pickerel

Bigmouth buffalo (sucker)
Black buffalo

Carp
Chub

Mississippi catfish
Yellow bullhead (catfish)

Eel
  Common European
  Common North
    American

Conger eel

Atlantic cod (scrod)[4]
Cusk
Haddock[4]
Pollack
Silver hake
Tomcod

Mullet
  Gray (striped)
  Silver
  White

Silversides (white bait)

Bass
  Black sea
  Oriental spotted
  Striped (rockfish)
Brown grouper (speckled
  hind)
Red Grouper (red hind)
White perch

Red snapper

Grunt
  Gray
  Common
  Yellow

Bass (black)
  Large-mouth (big-
    mouth)
  Small-mouth
  Spotted
Bluegill
Long-eared sunfish
Pumpkinseed sunfish

Pike (wall-eye)
Yellow perch

Tilefish

Bluefish

Amberjack
Jack mackerel
Pompano

Dolphin fish

Atlantic croaker
Freshwater drumfish
King whiting
Silver perch
Weakfish

Porgy (scup)

Mackerel Family
Albacore
Atlantic bonito
Bluefish tuna
Chile bonito
Mackerel
  Atlantic
  Frigate
  King
  Spanish
Skipjack tuna

Marlin
Sailfish

Swordfish

Butterfish
Harvestfish

California halibut
Southern flounder
Summer flounder

Atlantic halibut
Pacific halibut
Winter flounder

European sole
Common sole
Turbot

Rosefish (ocean perch)

Sea robin (sea tag)

Puffer

American bullfrog
European bullfrog

Diamondback terrapin

Green turtle

Snapping turtle

Rattlesnake
  Eastern diamondback
  Western diamondback

American alligator

Mallard duck
Greylag goose

Partridge (ruffed grouse)
Prairie chicken

Peacock
  Egg

Domestic chicken (Indian
  pheasant)
  Egg
  Liver
Cornish hen
Domestic pheasant
Peafowl
Quail

Domestic goose
  Egg
Domestic duck
  Egg

Guinea fowl

Turkey
  Egg

Dove
Pigeon (squab)

Opossum

Belgian hare
Domestic rabbit
Eastern cottontail
Jackrabbit

[4]Cod and haddock look and taste alike and cost the same; at times one may be substituted for the other.

Snowshoe rabbit
Western cottontail

Domestic guinea pig

Prairie dog
Squirrel (fox, red, gray)
Woodchuck

Beaver

Whale
(several families)

Porpoise

Dolphin

Wolf

Bear
Black
Brown
Grizzly
Polar

Raccoon

Lion
Tiger

Walrus

Sea lion

Common seal

Elephant
Asiatic
African

Horse

Pig (pork)
Bacon
Gelatin
Ham
Lard

Hippopotamus

Camel

Llama

American Elk
Caribou
Reindeer
European red deer

White-tailed deer
Moose

Giraffe
Antelope

Bovine Family
African buffalo
American bison
Brahman
Domestic cattle (beef)
Butter
Cheese[5]
Cow's milk[5]
Gelatin
Liver[5]
Other organs
Veal (young cattle)
Goat
Cheese[5]
Goat's milk[5]
Sheep
Lamb
Mutton

PLANTS: BIOLOGICALLY RELATED GROUPS

Agar[6]
Kelp
Seaweeds

Fungi
Molds in cheese
Mushroom
Truffle
Yeast[7]
Baker's
Brewer's

Florida arrowroot
(zamia)

Honey[8]

Grass Family
Bamboo shoots

Barley
Malt
Maltose
Rye
Wheat
Bran
Bulgur
Farina
Flour
Gluten
Graham
Patent
Semolina
Whole wheat
Wheat germ—Oil
Triticale

Millet
Oats
Oatmeal
Rice
Flour
Wild rice
Sugarcane
Molasses
Raw sugar
Sorghum
Grain
Syrup
Corn
Hominy grits
Corn oil
Cornmeal
(continued)

[5] Cheese, milk, and liver come from the same animal, but they are sufficiently different from the meat (muscle tissue), in the allergic sense, that they should be tried on a two-day rotation.

[6] Agar has been used in laxatives.

[7] Antibiotics are made from molds.

[8] Honey comes from different species of flowers.

Grass Family *(cont.)*
Corn sugar / syrup /
sweetener
Dextrose (Glucose)
Cornstarch
Popcorn
Vitamin C[9]

Chinese water chestnut

Palm Family
Coconut
Oil
Meal
Sago palm
Starch[9] (vitamin C)[9]
Date palm
Dates
Sugar
Palm cabbage

Taro
Poi
Malanga

Pineapple

Lily Family
Aloe
Asparagus
Chives
Garlic
Leek
Onion
Ramp
Shallot
Yucca

Fiji arrowroot (tacca)

Sarsaparilla

Yam
American
Chinese
Indian
Tropical

Banana
Plantain
Arrowroot (musa)

Saffron
Orris root

Ginger Family
Ginger
Turmeric
Cardamom
East Indian arrowroot
(Curcuma)

West Indian arrowroot
(maranta)

Vanilla

Black pepper (white)[10]

Walnut Family
Hickory
Pecan
Walnut
Black
English
White (butternut)

Birch Family
Filbert
Hazelnut
Oil of birch

Beechnut
Chestnut

Mulberry Family
Breadfruit
Fig
Hop
Mulberry

Macadamia nut

Buckwheat Family
Buckwheat
Garden sorrel
Rhubarb

Goosefoot Family
Beet[11]
Sugar beet (beet sugar)
Swiss chard
Lamb's quarters
Spinach
Tampala

Olive
Green
Olive oil
Ripe

American pawpaw
Custard apple

Nutmeg
Mace

Laurel Family
Avocado
Bay leaf
Cinnamon
Sassafras (file)

Chinese lotus

Poppy seed

Mustard Family
Broccoli[11]
Brussels sprouts
Cabbage
Cauliflower
Celery cabbage
Collards
Kale
Kohlrabi
Chinese cabbage
Horseradish
Mustard
Greens
Seed
Radish
Rutabaga
Turnip
Watercress

Caper

[9] Vitamin C is manufactured from corn. A small number of corn-sensitive individuals do not tolerate this form of vitamin C, and the sago-palm product (Nutricology Laboratory) is an excellent source of this nutrient. Another type of vitamin C is prepared from potato. Vitamin C is also manufactured from grape sugar in Europe.

[10] Peppercorns have black skins. Whole ground pepper is black. If the skins are removed first, white pepper results.

[11] These foods are very closely related and may be tolerated on alternate days by some individuals, but for others they must be considered to be identical in the allergic sense.

Pomegranate

Brazil nut

Berry Family
Blackberry[11, 12]
Boysenberry
Dewberry
Loganberry
Youngberry
Raspberry (black, red)
Rose hips
Strawberry
Wineberry

Apple Family
Apple[12]
  {Butter / Juice / Sauce
  {Cider
  Pectin
  Vinegar
Crabapple
Loquat
Pear
Quince

Plum Family
Almond[12]
Apricot
Cherry
Nectarine
Peach
Plum
  Prune

Currant
Gooseberry

Legume Family
Alfalfa
{Bush
{Jack
{Kidney
{Navy   } Bean[11]
{Pinto
{String
{Broad   } Bean[11]
{Windsor
Carob
Clover
Coumarin
Fenugreek

Flaxseed
Gum acacia
Gum tragacanth
Lentil
Licorice
Lima bean
Mung (sprout)
Pea (sweet / green)
Black-eyed pea
  (Cow pea)
Chick pea
  (Garbanzo)
  (Spanish pea)
Peanut
Pigeon pea
Soybean
  Flour
  Grits
  Lecithin
  Milk
  Oil
  Tofu
Snow pea
Tamarind
Tonka bean

Citrus Family
Angostura
Citron
Grapefruit
Kumquat
Lemon
Lime
Mandarin orange
  Tangerine
Orange

Barbados cherry
  (Acerola)

{Cassava (meal)
{Tapioca
{ (Brazilian arrowroot)
{Yucca

Nut
Lychee

Cashew Family
Cashew
Mango

Pistachio

Sugar maple
  Maple sugar
  Maple syrup

Grape
  Cream of tartar
  Muscadine
  Raisin
  Slipskin
  Vinegar (wine)
  Wine (brandy,
    champagne)

Cocoa
  Chocolate
Cola nut

Cottonseed
  Meal
  Oil
Okra

Kiwi fruit
  (Chinese gooseberry)

Tea

Passion fruit

Papaya

Clove Family
Allspice
Clove
Eucalyptus
Guava

Arrowroot

Carrot Family
Angelica
Anise
Caraway
Carrot
Celeriac
Celery
Chervil
Coriander
Cumin
Dill
Fennel
Parsley
Parsnip

[12] The rose family has three major divisions—the berry, apple, and plum groups. These groups differ enough from each other to be considered separate families in constructing individual diets.

Ginseng
  American
  Asian

Heath Family
Bearberry
Blueberry
Cranberry
Huckleberry
Wintergreen

Persimmon
  American[*]
  Oriental

Chicle

Nightshade Family
Eggplant
Ground cherry
Pepper[11]
  Garden (green/bell/
    sweet)
  Cayenne
  Chili
  Paprika
  Pimiento
Potato (white/Irish)[9]
Tobacco—not a food but
    is chewed
Tomato

Mint Family
Apple mint
Basil
Bergamot
Chia seed
Clary
Chinese artichoke
Horehound
Horse mint
Hyssop
Lavender
Lemon balm
Marjoram
Oregano
Pennyroyal

Peppermint
Rosemary
Sage
Savory
Spearmint
Thyme
Water mint

Sweet potato

Comfrey

Sesame
  Oil
  Seeds
  Tahini
  Butter

Coffee

Elderberry

Gourd Family
Chinese preserving
  melon
Cucumber
Melon[11]
  Cantaloupe
  Casaba
  Crenshaw
  Honeydew
  Musk
  Persian
  Spanish
Indian gherkin
Pumpkin
  (seeds, meal)[11]
Summer squash
  Crookneck, yellow
  Pattypan
  Spaghetti
  Zucchini
Large pumpkin[11]
Winter squash
  Acorn
  Butternut
  Hubbard
  Turban

Watermelon

Lettuce Family
Absinthe
Artichoke
  Common
  Jerusalem (flour)
Burdock Root
Cardoon
Chamomile
Chicory
Coltsfoot
Costmary
Dandelion
Endive
Escarole
French endive
  (Witloof chicory)
Goldenrod
Lettuce
Romaine
Safflower oil
Salsify
  (Oyster plant)
Santolina
Scolymus
  (Spanish oyster)
Scozzonera
  (Black salsify)
Southernwood
Sunflower
  Meal
  Oil
  Seed
Tansy
Tarragon
Vermouth
Wormwood

Juniper (gin)
Pine nut

New Zealand spinach

Cactus pear (prickly)

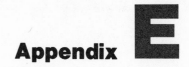

EAT ANYWHERE (IN YOUR DIET) FOODS

The following foods may be substituted for any offending foods that you must remove, at least temporarily, from your diet. The "Eat Anywhere Foods" may be used in any of the diets in this book. It is not necessary for you to look up their food families in the "Food Family Checklist," because these foods are unrelated to any other foods in your diet; they are the only members in their respective food families. Just remember not to repeat any one of them at intervals of less than four days.

PLANT KINGDOM

Fruit

Acerola cherry
Chinese gooseberry
  (Kiwi berry)
Currant
Elderberry
Grape (raisin)
Kiwi fruit
Lychee nut
Olive
Papaya
Passion fruit
Persimmon
Pineapple
Pomegranate
Prickly pear (cactus)

Nut/Seed

Brazil nut
Chestnut[1]
Chinese water chestnut
Flaxseed
Lychee nut
Macadamia nut
Pine nut (pinyon)
Poppy seed
Sesame

Spice/Flavor

Black pepper
Caper
Honey
Maple sugar/syrup
Saffron
Vanilla

Vegetable

Arrowroot[2]
New Zealand spinach
Sweet potato[3]
Tapioca
Yam

---

[1] Chestnuts are related to beechnuts, but beechnuts are not very often available and you can have chestnuts "anywhere" if there are no beechnuts in your diet.

[2] There are many kinds of arrowroot that are not related to each other. If you can determine the exact kinds that are available in your local stores, it is possible to eat a different kind of arrowroot every day of your four- to seven-day rotation cycle.

[3] Yams and sweet potatoes are from different families, but they are often confused or mislabeled in markets. Sweet potatoes have thin skins and look like new potatoes. Ask for help from the produce man.

ANIMAL KINGDOM

Mammals	Birds	Fish
Antelope	Partridge	Anchovy
Bear	Peacock	Bluefish
Beaver	Turkey	Carp
Elephant	Wild duck	Catfish
Hippopotamus		Dolphin
Horse	**Amphibians**	Eel
Lion	Frogs' legs	Mullet
Llama	Diamondback terrapin	Porgy (scup)
Opossum	Green turtle	Porpoise
Pork	Snapping turtle	Puffer
Rabbit		Red snapper
Squirrel	**Reptiles**	Sea robin
Whale	Rattlesnake	Shark (maco and others)
		Smelt
Shellfish	**Snails**	Sturgeon
Abalone	Octopus	Swordfish
Clam	Squid	Tarpon
Cockle		Tilefish
Oyster		Lake whitefish
Crab		
Lobster		
Shrimp		

NOTE: There are many kinds of game meat and game birds available for a rotation of high-protein foods for individuals who cannot tolerate the usual high-protein foods. Czimers Food, Inc., of Lockport, IL, has a very broad selection that they will ship frozen: RR #1, Box 285, 60441. Send for catalog.

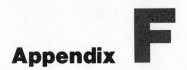

COMMON SOURCES OF HIDDEN FOOD ALLERGENS

Baker's Yeast

Barbecue Sauce
Brandy
Buttermilk
Catsup
Cheese
Citrus fruit juices, frozen
    or canned
Cottage Cheese
Gin
Horseradish
Leavening
Malted Products
Mayonnaise
Mushrooms
Olives
Pickles
Rum
Sauerkraut
Vinegar
Vodka
Whiskey
Wine

Brewer's Yeast

B Vitamins
Beer
Wine

Chlorine

Anything with City Water
Coffee
Juices
Soda
Tea
Water

Corn

Aspirin
Bacon
Baking Mixes
Baking Powder
Beer
Bleached Flours
Carbonated Beverages
Chewing Gum
Cough Syrups
"Cream of . . ." Cereals
Glue on back of Stamps
    and Envelopes
Gravies
Instant Coffee
Instant Teas
Salad Dressings
Talcums
Toothpaste
Vanilla
Vitamins
Zest

Dust

Wine

ECP, Tetracycline, Other Antibiotics

Beef
Chicken
Eggs
Seafood (fish markets and
    grocery stores treat
    their ice with
    antibiotics)
Turkey

Egg

Albumin
Baked Goods
Bouillons
Hamburger Mix
Hollandaise Sauce
Ice Cream
Noodles
Ovaltine
Pancake Flours
Pretzels
Soups
Tartar Sauce
Wine

Food Colorings

Butter
Certain Fruits (e.g.,
    oranges)
Fruit Juices
Margarine
Mouthwash
Processed Meats
Soft Drinks
Toothpaste

Formaldehyde

Cosmetics, especially nail
    polish and lipstick
Milk
Shampoo
Soap
Tea

Milk	Mold	Soy
Au Gratin Dishes	Cheese	Baby Formulas
Baked Goods	Nuts	Breads
Bologna	Wine	Candy
Butter		Cereals
Cocoa Drinks		Ice Creams
Doughnuts		Lecithin[1]
Gravies		Lunch Meats
Hamburgers		Margarine
Ice Cream		Mayonnaise (label may
Junket		only say vegetable
Meat Loaf		oil; you must inquire)
Ovaltine		Meat Extender
Sauces		Milk Substitutes
Sausages		Plastics, especially in
Sherbet		Ford Cars
Soups		Pork Link Sausages
Waffles		Salad Dressings
Whey		Sauces

---

[1]Lecithin is an emulsifier in food and a stabilizer in leaded gasoline.

Sugar	Wheat
Beer	Barley Malt
Catsup	Beer
Cereals	Bologna
Infant Formulas	Bouillon
Mayonnaise	Bran
Mouthwash	Candy
Salad Dressings	Crackers
Salt	Cream of Wheat
Toothpaste	Farina
Wine	Flours
	Gin
	Gluten
	Graham
	Gravies
	Hamburger
	Ice Cream (thickening agents)
	Licorice
	Liverwurst
	Macaroni
	Matzohs
	Mayonnaise
	Ovaltine
	Pancake Mix
	Pepper (synthetic)
	Postum
	Puddings
	Pumpernickel
	Rye Bread
	Soups
	Soy Sauce
	Vitamin E
	Wheat Germ
	Whiskey
	Yeasts (some)

SUGGESTED READING

BOOKS

Dickey, Lawrence D., M.D., ed. *Clinical Ecology.* Springfield, Ill.: Charles C. Thomas, 1976.

Forman, Robert. *How to Control Your Allergies.* New York: Larchmont Books, 1979.

Golos, Natalie, and Golbits, Frances Golos, with Leighton, Frances Spatz. *Coping with Your Allergies.* New York: Simon & Schuster, 1979.

Hosen, Harris, M.D. *Clinical Allergy (Based on Provocative Testing).* (Available through Dr. Hosen's office, Proctor Street, Port Arthur, Texas.)

Mandell, Fran Gare. *Dr. Mandell's Allergy Free Cookbook.* New York: Pocket Books, 1981.

Mandell, Marshall, M.D., and Scanlon, Lynne Waller. *Dr. Mandell's 5-Day Allergy Relief System.* New York: Pocket Books, 1980.

Mandell, Marshall, M.D. *Dr. Mandell's Lifetime Arthritis Relief System.* New York: Coward, McCann and Geoghegan, 1983.

Nikel, D., and Pfeiffer, G. O. *Household Environments and Chronic Illness.* Springfield, Ill.: Charles C. Thomas, 1980.

Philpott, W. H., and Kalita, D. *Brain Allergies.* New Canaan, CT: Keats, 1980.

Randolph, Theron G., M.D., and Moss, Ralph W., Ph.D. *An Alternate Approach to Allergies.* New York: Lippincott & Crowell, 1980.

Randolph, Theron G., M.D. *Human Ecology and Susceptibility to the Chemical Environment.* Springfield, Ill.: Charles C. Thomas, 1962.

Rapp, Doris J., M.D. *Allergies and Your Family*. New York: Sterling, 1980.

Rinkel, H. J., M.D.; Randolph, T. G., M.D.; and Zeller, M., M.D. *Food Allergy*. Springfield, Ill.: Charles C. Thomas, 1951. (Available from the New England Foundation for Allergic and Ecologic Disease, 3 Brush Street, Norwalk, Conn. 06850.)

Travis, Nick, and Holaday, Ruth. *The Body Wrecker*. Amarillo: Don Quixote Publishing, 1981.

Williams, Roger J., Ph.D. *Nutrition Against Disease; Environmental Prevention*. New York: Putnam, 1971.

Zamm, Alfred F., M.D., with Gannon, Robert. *Why Your House May Endanger Your Health*. New York: Simon & Schuster, 1980.

SCIENTIFIC PAPERS

Randolph, Theron G., "The Alternation of the Symptoms of Allergy and Those of Alcoholism and Certain Mental Disturbances." *Journal of Laboratory and Clinical Medicine* 40:932, 1952.

Randolph, Theron G., M.D. "Food Addiction; Addictive Eating and Drinking." *Quarterly Journal of Studies on Alcoholism* 17:195–224, 1956.

Mandell, Marshall, M.D., and Conte, Anthony, M.D. "The Role of Allergy in Arthritis, Rheumatism and Polysymptomatic Cerebral, Visceral and Somatic Disorders: A Double-Blind Study." *J. Int. Acad. of Preventive Med.* Vol. VII, no. 2 (1982).

Mandell, Marshall, M.D. "The Diagnostic Value of Therapeutic Fasting and Food Ingestion Tests in a Controlled Environment: Chronic Multiple-System Cerebro-Viscerosomatic Ailments Demonstrated to Be Unsuspected and Unrecognized Food Allergies. *J. Int. Acad. of Metabology* IV, no. 1 (1975).